Teach in the Positive Circle

Teach in the Positive Circle

Creating Opportunities for Growth and Reflection

Julie West

ROWMAN & LITTLEFIELD
Lanham • Boulder • New York • London

Published by Rowman & Littlefield
An imprint of The Rowman & Littlefield Publishing Group, Inc.
4501 Forbes Boulevard, Suite 200, Lanham, Maryland 20706
www.rowman.com
86-90 Paul Street, London EC2A 4NE, United Kingdom

Copyright © 2022 by Julie West

All rights reserved. No part of this book may be reproduced in any form or by any electronic or mechanical means, including information storage and retrieval systems, without written permission from the publisher, except by a reviewer who may quote passages in a review.

British Library Cataloguing in Publication Information Available

Library of Congress Cataloging-in-Publication Data Available

ISBN 978-1-4758-6574-5 (cloth)
ISBN 978-1-4758-6575-2 (pbk.)
ISBN 978-1-4758-6576-9 (electronic)

To all the hardworking educators—I see you, and you do make a difference daily in our children's future destinies.

Contents

Preface ix
Acknowledgments xiii
Introduction xv
Chapter 1: The Start of Something New 1
Chapter 2: Relationships and Connections 5
Chapter 3: Diving Deep into Relationships 9
Chapter 4: Self-Awareness 15
Chapter 5: Professionalism 19
Chapter 6: Intentions and Best Practices for Learning 23
Chapter 7: Lesson Preparation 25
Chapter 8: New Mindset and Self-Care 29
Chapter 9: The Pessimist Syndrome 33
Chapter 10: One, Two, Three: Evaluator and Me 37
Chapter 11: Life outside of School 41
Chapter 12: New Teacher Growth in the First Year 45
Chapter 13: Teacher Retention 49
Chapter 14: Administrator: Friend or Foe? 53
Chapter 15: Roll Out and Monitor 59
Chapter 16: Management 63
Chapter 17: Scenarios 69

Chapter 18: Feedback	79
Chapter 19: Parent Communication	83
Chapter 20: Parent–Teacher Conference	89
Chapter 21: Midyear Rejuvenation	93
Chapter 22: Student Engagement	95
Chapter 23: Gratitude and Educators	99
Chapter 24: End of the Year	103
Chapter 25: The Last Hour: Now What?	105
Chapter 26: Final Thoughts	107
Epilogue	115
Bibliography	119
About the Author	121

Preface

According to almost all research, student–teacher relationships considerably influence teacher effectiveness and student achievement. For example, John Hattie states, "It is teachers who have created positive teacher–student relationships which are more likely to have above-average effects on student achievement."

A few years back, I was approached by a valued administrator with the question, "Why are your test scores one of the highest in our district?" I clearly stated it was all based around relationships. In my experience, it was very accurate. Students would gain trust and respect the more time I invested in them. They seem to set higher goals and work harder with encouragement and belief in them.

I would get to know my students and drive the passion inside of them. I would enter the room on the first day of school, tell them my name, and proceed with telling them they were in the "gifted class." I would then say, "If you should not be in the gifted class, you can leave at this time." Every year, I would have students looking at each other back and forth. They would question if they should leave, but no one ever stood up and walked out. So, I would then explain to students, each had a gift, and it would be the goal as a class this year to find the "special gift." We would work as partners all year to discover those individual gifts and celebrate. We did a lot of celebrations in our classroom.

I strived to break what seemed to be a negative, harsh, and unhappy education cycle. The belief in my classroom was of very high expectations for all students. Students knew what behavior and hard work consisted of from day one. Each one pushed themselves to reach their own goals and make achievements. Somehow, educators oftentimes fall into the comfort zone of how one grew up in education. Often when things become problematic in the classroom, teachers model the behavior they grew up watching. Unfortunately, this could mean a harsher style than they truly needed to communicate. If you were a part of the lecture era, it might not be as easy to become part of the technology and engagement era. Our focus must always be on relationships, high expectations, and student mastery. Our most significant understanding of education is that relationships feed us daily. We must nurture our relationships with people. Education must be fun and curious—we must lighten up and enjoy our journey.

It is easy to form the belief that our world is full of negativity; we must learn to affirm and celebrate each other. Everyone is just searching to feel a sense of belonging somewhere, even as adults. I soon realized this when I accepted a job as Student Achievement Coordinator—gaining an understanding early on that teachers need affirmations daily, much like students. Adults want to feel respected and have a sense of belonging. I worked side by side with teachers and gave ongoing feedback to drive new results in their practice.

I began to realize that our district needed to invest more energy in new teachers. Early on in education, I had been a part of a new teacher academy. A sagacious woman named Marsha Mason, a wonderful mentor, had led the academy. She was authentic about the expectations of our first year. I was truly grateful for such transparency. It was a place where everyone felt safe to ask difficult questions.

A model to support the knowledge needed to conquer the first year, full of questions and fears, came to fruition. A partner joined in, and with the support of our district, we worked long hours to support and retain our new teachers. It would be an academy model where new teachers would come together once a month to learn and gain support by studying different topics. Our district soon found that educators were striving to feel united and part of a particular group to relate and communicate comfortably. As a result, these teachers would be themselves and feel a little imperfect at times. Soon our findings showed that new teachers formed a sense of belonging through these meetings, and their achievement grew. They seemed to have an investment in the district indeed.

As time went by, one could see the connections happening. Relationships were starting to build, and transparency was rearing its face. Many tears appeared as we traveled through our journey together. Lessons learned above all that these new teachers just wanted to be listened to and supported. Never believe that a positive relationship can't change your life; build them, practice them, and reflect on them.

Many education lessons have been added to my practitioner toolbox through different exhilarating experiences. One belief is that this is the result of a "wanderlust soul"—traveling as a flight attendant for ten years and working with many different personality types while connecting to many multicultural people played a significant role. Meeting many famous personalities on my journey led to deep conversations; each takeoff was a differentiated learning experience. These experiences molded the being of my existence into an upbeat, grateful, and adventurous personality.

Acknowledgments

To my husband, Eric, and children Brittanee and Bailey. Thank you for always encouraging my dreams. To my exceptional parents for listening to ongoing silly stories when I was young and celebrating each one. Thank you for always encouraging me to write. You truly believed I could do anything I set my mind to.

A sincere thank you to Tom Koerner and Kira Hall for making the publishing process a seamless success. Thank you to Professor John Hattie, Dr. Melanie Magee, and Dr. Georgeanne Warnock for ongoing educational support. My C&I team, Mrs. R, Edna, GG, Deanna, Camille, Monica, Gabi, Amy, Jinnifer, Brenda, Alison, Dr. Trimble, Julie Fisher, Dr. Polk, Melissa Nichols, Ms. Cooper, Melodie (friends—Kelly and Jeremy), and Terrell ISD for all the inspirational beliefs and laughs along the way. To my Alaska family and friends for the cultural experience and new lifestyle. To Rockwall ISD family and friends, Jennifer, true friend and mentor, Jill for all the third-grade laughs, and especially Marsha Mason, my new teacher mentor, for the first step in my passion for education.

Introduction

What does it mean to be a part of the positive circle? The circle represents every relationship that an educator will encounter throughout a lifetime. The circle is oneself and the positive energy; it encompasses. When the circle centers around growth and reflection it will begin to radiate self-confidence and optimism.

Positive relationships are a challenge in this ever-changing world we live in today but even more so in education. Teaching is a heroic profession. Teachers have a tremendous influence on the lives of not only their students but their entire families. In addition, they have the massive responsibility of educating future generations and enabling them to recognize their potential and strive to achieve it. Nevertheless, despite their significance in society, they are compensated relatively meagerly. We will uncover what allows each individual to sign up for this task and how they survive and even thrive.

Teachers must navigate relationships with students, parents, administrators, and peers while planning lessons, managing student behavior, complying with educational standards, satisfying administrators' demands, and promoting career growth. It is a challenge; teachers must have the proper support and preparation to overcome the many obstacles and become the inspirational role models that all children need and deserve.

Teachers will begin to understand how to become the light in all aspects of education and the true meaning of gratitude—as well as continue to understand that priority is the value of every relationship at all times. It will take much work for the mind, body, and spirit. Some will call it a mission, a calling, or even destiny.

Reflections will be enlightening whether the person is entering the educational field as a brand-new teacher or a seasoned teacher open to change. So, gather around and get comfortable—discovering new attitudes and approaches to staying positive in education will soon become very clear.

It is a matter of understanding the key ingredient: relationships. Staying in the positive circle allows formation of successful relationships and seeing the best in everyone and everything. It will be a time to gaze at the inner self as well. When facing challenges, one will learn to have the strength and a sense of remaining calm. Reflections will occur on how to look to a bright future and not linger in the past.

In many studies throughout history, positive reinforcement in education is highly effective with every daily interaction. Specific examples will be provided and practiced effectively throughout this text to gain the support needed for daily success. When drawn to the negative side, one will be equipped with the tools to quickly travel back to the positive circle, learning of specific strategies to apply when one gets frustrated, beaten down, and broken, and most of all, wanting to give up.

The positive circle will allow the teacher to celebrate and explore issues of concern with respect—and also to allow children a place to address issues that may distress them in a safe atmosphere. It will provide a structured mechanism for solving a problem where all participants have an equal footing. Teachers will understand how to remain the light. Detailed examples will transform common classroom management issues into positive experiences and interactions. In addition, the reflection on classroom culture, diversity, and expectations will allow further growth and successful implementation.

One will begin to honestly believe the mantra that teachers can bring positivity to every situation. Remember, as one proceeds with the journey, the circle remains open at all times. An open heart, open-mindedness, and openness to all experiences will allow every relationship to have value and flourish.

The educators' end goal will evolve into quality work and stay in a culture of feeling heard, maintaining health, and keeping positive support throughout the first few years and an entire career. This step-by-step educational guide focusing on positivity, growth, and reflection will allow for lifelong happiness in and out of education.

Here is the first set of reflections:

- What is your why?
- What do your decision-making skills look like?
- How do you understand one's truth?
- How do you choose to make the best of every situation?
- How do you shift the focus to encountering failure as a lesson of learning?
- How do you move on quickly to the positive?
- How do you learn that perspective is a daily choice to identify and nurture?
- How does teaching yourself to focus on the good instead of the bad support mental health?
- How do you approach feedback in a positive manner?

Chapter 1

The Start of Something New

It is only a few weeks before school begins. The air is thick with intense heat and long summer nights. Families are enjoying last-minute vacations, swimming in pools, and late-night ice cream runs. However, it looks pretty different for an educator come early July. Educators begin to gain access into schools to set up classrooms—everything from putting together furniture, to placing the fabric on bulletin boards, to creating an excellent classroom library.

The first-year teacher has made it through final classes, resumés, a rigorous interview, and many background checks, all completed with extreme detail. Contracts are signed, and reality begins to set in. They are frantically setting up a classroom and balancing a social life all on a personal budget—a daily reminder that a first-year educator's paycheck will not arrive until late September. Due to the new job, some have moved away from their parents and entered new cities, states, or homes.

The body and mind are already mentally and physically exhausted from trying to process all the information. Daily, one's heart beats rapidly, breath quickens, and muscles become tense. The feeling of multi-tasking has never been more intense. But, above all, teachers fear that their education toolbox is not very advanced. Worry begins to loom over them daily, even after the first student enters the classroom.

Great news, it is time to develop some strategies for success. First, new teachers must chunk out what is necessary at the moment. The beginning of the year checklist will allow a new teacher to view specific priorities and focus on the essential needs at hand.

Begin to be cautious from the first day you enter the building. Watch for the many negative triggers and know that the daily chronic work stress can quickly lead to burnout. Some signs to watch for daily are feeling overemotional, overwhelming exhaustion, and losing personal balance. It is challenging to stay positive without feeling prepared. That first day of school can feel intimidating. Walk in the building the first day feeling confident and ready for whatever comes with these tips.

Checklist Prior to Day One:

- Prepare home life; examples—childcare, laundry, weekly meetings.
- Pack a lunch in advance.
- Make a plan to arrive early for the first three days; a suggestion might be the entire year. A good note is to arrive 45 minutes to an hour early, allowing for anything extra that may arise.
- Plan the first day of school outfit—lay it out, so you are ready to hit the ground running.
- Do not forget to set the alarm (not that you will sleep at all).
- Unforeseen circumstances—parking for the teacher.
- Overplan for the first day. (Plan the first day getting-to-know-student activities—remember, the relationship is everything!)
- Review student roster—check for all updates; students do not want to be left out.
- Know the first-day procedures from administrators, specifically paperwork.
- Put together your daily schedule, plan to arrive at lunch on time, special classes, and dismissal.
- Check yourself of all student accommodations.
- Review the curriculum plan—take a look at the year at a glance document provided by the district. Then, create a plan for the first three weeks of instruction. Next, practice this plan and time how long it takes to perform.

Suggestions:

- Learn your way around the school—get a map, if needed.
- Plan a seating chart for the first day (if you plan to allow students to sit where they would like, make sure to have a plan for any disruptions).
- Get a calendar ready (faculty meetings, professional learning committees, agendas, and much more).
- Be prepared with a selection of books to read. (Culturally appropriate books provide that sense of community from the start.)
- Create a self-plan for you and students to be flexible, innovative, and listening.
- Create high expectations from the beginning with an accountability process in place.
- Define the routines for the classroom. (Examples to consider include sharpening pencils, turning in work, asking for help.) What does the plan entail?
- How will students practice when done incorrectly?

- Know the attendance policy. If you do not know, ask someone. Ensure attendance is taken daily and on time; one suggestion might be to set reminders such as a timer.
- How will students get home on the first day? What are the school's dismissal procedures?
- Create policies for restroom breaks. Which bathrooms do they use? Will students travel alone? What are the specific procedures for the building routine?
- Develop a system for communicating with parents or caregivers on the first day of school.

Reflections:

- Are plans in place before the first day of school?
- Are you open minded and flexible?
- How will you ensure success on the student's first day?

STORY TIME

One incident in which a new teacher was very well planned and prepared for the first day. She had followed all the tips from top to bottom. The entire checklist had been reviewed many times. Unfortunately, it ended up backfiring when entering the building and suddenly realizing toilet paper was dangling from the back of the new teacher's pants. Even the best-laid plan can go awry. Sometimes all you can do is laugh and check yourself in the mirror. Remember, tomorrow is a new day.

Chapter 2

Relationships and Connections

In jaunting through an unknown territory of life, most of us prefer to navigate with someone. When we connect to others through all aspects of our lives, everything seems more valuable. One must take time to invest and become resilient in relationships, and over time we will find our most remarkable selves.

The priority in the first year is to value and nurture each new relationship. Forming healthy relationships takes time, trust, and consistency. Therefore, it is necessary to be compassionate, kind, and merciful. Once new teachers realize that all individuals should be valued, relationships will form authentic connections.

The relationship with new teachers travels through many territories. First, a connection with an immediate team will occur. Before school starts, take the initiative to meet and get to know each other. Learning about each other's interests and lives can achieve a simple kind of connection. If people begin to understand each other, more reflection, trust, and empathy will withstand the rough times. Once school professional development begins, it will foster and grow through team-building activities that support forming relationships and include the rest of the faculty.

Connections will continue through planning, collaborating, and listening to each other. Periodically, stop and ask: What is working? What is not working? Is there a good balance? Learning how to trust a new team and depend upon them can be difficult. One idea is to find a "work friend," or mentor, one you can go to when things become complicated. Another option is to find a collaborative thinking partner with whom to hash out ideas and plans. While navigating day-to-day life, the work friend or mentor can help build beautiful memories and aid in difficult situations.

In addition, at times, sharing experiences will enable others to see and understand the background or culture that brought one to education. Perhaps give a small "happy" to make a teammate's day—possibly a tiny note, coffee, chocolate, or just a listening ear. In education, a thinking partner will go a long way. Often, they will inspire innovation through one's questioning or thinking. In addition, the new teacher will find they can support and balance stress as a team much more successfully than alone.

However, sometimes a teammate will find a personality difficult. It will take work, dedication, practice, trust, and understanding to form a positive team. Do not bring the ego to the table. Remember empathy daily and that everyone involved is crucial for the greater purpose. If we see that a relationship needs work, communicate until the situation comes to a resolution. Do not allow matters to build up and fester.

Daily reminders to utilize the perspective that all teammates are doing their best and that all parties will make mistakes will allow flexibility in the workplace. Reflect and ask, is one making snap judgments or genuinely listening to the team's concerns?

Work to speak in kind responses and forgive minor incidents within individual relationships. Listening can be a powerful skill that shows much respect. When the team gives equal conversation time, a new teacher will feel comfortable and empowered to share their perspective. Often a new educator has excellent ideas to share but can be guarded because of doubt and insecurity. Sometimes a veteran teacher will not need to provide the answer. Often all that is needed is encouragement and general guidance. Entering conversations in the correct mindset will allow creative ideas to transpire.

Most of all, let go of the grudges and resentments. Opposing issues will arise, and it may be needed to seek out support. Work must be a place of safety and a location to maintain and express oneself. So, an important goal to keep in mind throughout a teaching career is to create a positive circle among these unique and new personalities.

New teachers will need to understand that education operates differently than any other occupation. Changes will occur daily, quarterly, and yearly with staff. There will be many different perspectives to maneuver, and multi-tasking will consume the new educator.

Fostering free-thinking and a reflective mindset can lead to early success. Sometimes, someone else's vision might be the best choice. Always place the student's views first when making any decision. If centering our positive circle around students is the priority, teachers will understand each other and develop empathy effectively. Sometimes it all comes down to just having manners and insisting others do likewise.

Truly being connected through tough times and stunning victories can be one of the greatest joys of education. In continuing to build a team culture, teachers can develop protocols to follow so everyone is respectful. Trust and collaboration with peers throughout the educational career will have a significant impact on student success. Realize early on that one must act as a trusted role model. Examples of this will be to honor commitments and provide some long-term thinking skills.

A teacher's positive energy will spread throughout the building. Little eyes will always watch the interaction classroom doorways, hallways, and in the cafeteria. Do not forget about office personnel, janitorial staff, cafeteria workers, and bus drivers. These crucial individuals play a prominent role in children's lives, too. Work to develop a positive, healthy relationship with these special people. Most importantly, show respect at all times.

Sometimes we may encounter differences, and we must strive to see eye to eye. Teamwork must mean solidarity, and one must aim to believe in the success of others. Teams often find that with experience and honoring opinions and diversity, they will perform better.

How will the team remain in the positive circle when encountering a difference, and how will one trek swiftly to the resolution?

Reflections:

- Is your mindset open to different perspectives?
- Are you listening and showing respect to the team?
- Are you celebrating diversity among the team?
- Are you being honest while being kind?
- Are you remaining calm in difficult situations?
- What changes will be needed personally?
- What is the plan if things are moving toward negativity?

STORY TIME

A teacher rapidly rounded the corner of the office after dropping off students at the gym. Suddenly, his feet begin to slide from a slippery waxed floor. Unable to catch his balance, a significant fall occurred. Suddenly, a piece of furniture with a plate came crashing down on the teacher's head. He looked up, with wide eyes, from the floor to see the principal hovering over, asking the question, "Are you okay?" The entire office staff came running out, providing support and comfort. The teacher got up slowly and regained composure. The situation turned from serious concern to comedy as laughter filled the air. The incident bonded them, and they all laughed for many years when recalling the incident.

Chapter 3

Diving Deep into Relationships

Close your eyes softly; for the next thirty seconds, consider the best moments in your lifetime (personal, professional, a revelation, or an exciting adventure). This activity has taken place at many professional workshops. The training places priority on reflecting on your personal life. It is easy to lose sight of these great moments and fall into a daily rut. We must not forget those best moments and begin thinking of teaching as one of those most significant moments. One of the biggest questions in life is figuring out who we are.

Next, we will dive deep into the two different relationships between ourselves and the students. In order to meet the needs of students, we must have a genuine understanding of ourselves. In beginning the journey of who we are, we must reflect. Take a moment and consider the following questions and jot down answers to discuss with a work friend or mentor:

- How do we begin to build an understanding of our feelings?
- Does one genuinely understand a healthy relationship with students?
- What techniques will teachers utilize as they begin to protect their energy?
- Does one understand what disturbs the energy and takes it to the negative side?
- Is one in a place where expectations may be too high?
- What does one need to release to prioritize growth with ease?
- How has one shown self-love today?
- How does one want students to perceive themselves as a person?
- What are one's beliefs about education and a growth mindset?
- How did one learn as a child?

When an understanding of how to love oneself occurs, it is genuinely easy to show others love. Educators must allow themselves to feel different emotions. So, first, learn how to regulate emotions and identify how genuine emotion feels. Then, accept every emotion, all of them. Be aware of wallowing and spending too much time in one emotion.

Positive energy in teaching is necessary at all times. There are many ways to gain knowledge about the kind of person we are and want to become. Find time for the quiet moments to know and understand yourself. One technique a new teacher can attempt is reflecting and journaling. Often, writing about the emotion will release the harmful components. The new teacher must remain open to different encounters. Remember to put good things and thoughts into the workday daily. Teachers should expect good things will happen daily. When you develop a good relationship with yourself daily, great things happen in the world.

Students want to feel love, hear love, and know love. Often a teacher is a primary source of learning this feeling correctly. Find different ways in which to continue to show students they are valued and loved. For example, making time for them and truly listening will support these emotions—as being fair and consistent in a safe atmosphere will support the feeling of love. These tips will also begin to bridge the struggle of classroom management. Sometimes little things make all the difference.

For example, it could just be taking an interest in what a student is doing in the extra-curricular life. Some specific ideas might be showing up at sporting events or practice, dance class, or band rehearsal. When the new educator is seen just making a simple gesture, it will be significant. Continue to build momentum upon interest, and the unique relationships will successfully grow.

Quality and caring teachers can significantly impact the success of children, particularly those coming from hardship and poverty. When students need direction, safety, confidence, and hope, school becomes this critical location. School provides children with enthusiasm for a different kind of future. An opportunity to remove themselves and move away from misery and misfortune. Some can break a cycle that has existed for many generations. A better tomorrow will occur for children through a caring teacher and quality education.

Considering each student's circumstances and the background will significantly guide a teacher in fulfilling their needs. In addition, with this information, teachers can anticipate behavioral problems, health problems, or family issues that may arise.

Students are entering the classroom who need serious social, and emotional learning support and guidance in their lives. In some cases, family members may be incarcerated, hospitalized, or otherwise unavailable to a child's needs. The problems will vary, and it is your job to stay alert and get the facts. When students have a sense of community, they will want to come to school and learn with joy. In addition, students will understand they need to take responsibility and own their actions.

Children are very skilled in hiding problems. Some will come to school hungry, cold, tired, beaten, and bruised. In some cases, the basic needs of children may not be met daily in life. When the educator begins to understand these unmet needs, a better understanding of the misbehavior will occur.

Some examples:

- food, water, sleep, clothing, and a safe shelter
- an activity like motor stimulation
- social and emotional connection with someone
- feeling heard or seen
- feeling respected
- feeling like they can achieve something

The homeless student does not show up and share all of their life problems on the first day. If teachers show genuine compassion and respect, they might begin to open up. Teachers' toolboxes begin to grow when they know and gain the understanding that these issues enter the doors daily. Academics may not always be the daily priority for every student. Children need to enter the new teacher's classroom understanding they are safe and will be taken care of every day with consistency.

One way to provide this is to create a classroom culture in which students feel supported and safe at all times. In a classroom culture, both the teacher and students should develop loyalty to the class and the group, resulting in a positive and productive atmosphere. Students in this kind of classroom act as if they are in one large family. It will provide the foundation for learning to occur successfully.

The mutual support system gives students teamwork skills they will need as an adult. At times, students will need to talk, write the problem down, or rest. So, what will the positive classroom circle center focus become? Reflect a moment on what stands out from the early days of being a student? What did the relationship look like with the adult? What kind of stimulating ideas and activities can you bring alive in the classroom? Who were the individuals that genuinely impacted your life? How will the goal be reached? What kind of books about emotions can be shared?

As educators, we must walk away from the comfort of the "old school" classroom. So many have been accustomed to this kind of educational process. The generation of students today needs to be taught differently. Gone are the days of the dictatorship and the teacher behind the desk, shouting orders. Instead, we need the creative teacher who tries new things and strives to reach all students. Do not be afraid to travel outside the safety of the known comfort zone.

Humor can often be the first line of defense. Having fun is not only okay; it is the only way to make it to retirement. Begin thinking of ways to be different in the classroom or fun events. Change the classroom energy by moving the activity to a fun book.

Laughing and reading for enjoyment are always fun. When new teachers can laugh at themselves, it allows more comfort and connection with students, and is fun and safe. The second example might be to tell a quick joke for a morning warm-up. Lastly, wearing something silly like funny glasses or a scarf. Teaching and learning should be full of gratification daily. Capture the students with things that make teaching fun, play special music, dance, play an instrument, do a cheer, and tell a story.

Students will enjoy gaining praise from the teacher. However, be cautious about giving authentic praise and being mindful of the correct times to use it. Well thought-out words will shift the possibilities and positivity. Students will feel that instant connection and deepen the bond for learning. So go ahead and enjoy planning and experimenting with all of these ideas.

Research has stated how it is imperative to take notice of positive behavior over negative behavior truly impacts kids. Modeling different perspectives should be a part of the classroom community. Remind students that teachers sometimes make mistakes; model a few along the way. Always separate the action from the child. When one implements check-in/check-outs and is present, it will support students' daily behavior changes. Remember, effective relationships will diminish off-task behavior and negatively prevent discipline.

Students who feel relationships at school are:

- More likely to come to school on time and miss fewer days
- More likely to feel good about themselves
- More likely to plan for a future of success

Students with feelings of closeness with their teacher have shown success. They strive for a better future and build a strong work ethic.

Students seem to:

- Work harder and retain information
- Spend more time trying and problem-solving
- Have more confidence in their abilities

To remain connected, educators must remain calm and reflective. It is effortless to be reactive and jump to a conclusion. These assumptions can cause communication obstacles, where one can judge or decide something without having all the facts; to reach unwarranted conclusions. It can very easily lead to harmful or rash decisions that can harm effective communication and positive relationships. We must work to not make decisions without first gathering all the information.

Reflections:

- How is the practice involving quality relationships evolving?
- Is the educator noticing if a child is tired, hungry, or in need?
- What needs to be changed?
- Have we had fun today with our practice?
- How will you enhance creativity and be a risk-taker daily? (It is hard to believe your ideas are worthy as a first-year teacher, but guess what? They are)
- How will you be positive and travel to the unknown?

STORY TIME

One fall day, a student wanted to stay and talk to a teacher during recess. The young teacher happened to have an off-duty that day. Instead of brushing the young boy off, she sat and listened. He began to tell the story of being stabbed by his mother years ago. The boy proceeded to show her the scars from the incident. He discussed the trauma and how the mother was now in jail. The young boy replied that he felt comfortable sharing something about himself. Holding back tears, he communicated that he had never been in a classroom where he felt safe. He thanked her for being a great teacher.

Chapter 4

Self-Awareness

Take a long look and begin to reflect and honestly know yourself. It is the center of the circle. You must face the facts for a few moments, and reality is sometimes brutal to swallow; the days and weeks will become prolonged, dark, and demanding. In this time, you will have to buckle up and find inner determination and more strength than ever thought. Here, you must choose to train those internal thoughts to stay clear, centered, and positive. It will be challenging, and it will take commitment and much work to prepare proper thoughts.

Work is and always will be stressful; teacher stress and anxiety are nothing new. One helpful recommendation is to meditate daily. Work at the connection with the team and school. Do not pull back and become a person on a lone island. Teaching is the kind of profession where we need others. You must remember, teachers will never be successful alone.

Sometimes you will start to hear the inner voice weeks into the new school year. It might feel like you are not good enough, like you are a failure. The inner voice might be saying you're in way over your head.

Do not allow these fears to get in the way of the goal. Remember, get past these by intentionally turning to positive thoughts and training the mind. The new teacher may encounter walking in the hallway and hearing other teachers yell at students during these long days. It might begin to deplete the positive energy. Focus the attention on blocking out the noise. Instead, find that quiet place and get in tune with the correct thoughts, not the negative ones.

Remain watchful of daily catastrophizing situations. Teachers and students often expect the worst without reason or logic. Honing into believing these thoughts will make days inevitably dreadful. Instead, recognize these thoughts and halt them before they can become cumbersome and then turn into a negative habit.

New teachers must seize the thoughts that brought them to this profession in the first place. It will take a lot of training and practice. Nevertheless, creating a community of trust, respect, and communication is crucial to create the best atmosphere for learning. Many begin to ask how a new teacher can begin to maximize their potential.

Unfortunately, some never will, not because they are lazy but because they do not understand how to reach it. One true thing is that educators are the most complex, hard-working people in the world. Often sight is lost because of inadequate training of thoughts and views. The reflective mindset must be at the forefront at all times. A better understanding of feelings may occur when writing down thoughts, and the balance will be more manageable. Journaling will often support in arranging distresses and difficulties. It will allow one to see day-to-day triggers. It can identify negative thoughts and shift and keep the balance of the positive circle.

You will begin to know yourself at a much deeper level. Take the time and read the journal entries and reflect on the emotions you have written down. Sometimes you will find a collection of good things to look at and share in no time at all. Then, begin to brainstorm ways you might need to adjust or reflect. Lists can be beneficial in keeping positive thoughts. If we do not honestly know ourselves and our students, we cannot succeed in our practice. Therefore, travel quickly back to exhibit, sustain, maintain, and reestablish when necessary.

Reflections:

- How will you tune in to the inner voice and build on positive daily thoughts? (Teaching can bring out negative thoughts; practice working at building the positive.)
- How will you find and connect with the right people—positive people? (You will meet many people who choose the right ones to gravitate to and make your tribe.)
- What intentions will be set to travel to the solution instead of dwelling on the problem? (It is easy to wallow in the problem; search and reflect—the solution will come.)
- How will you enhance creativity and be a risk-taker daily? (It is hard to believe your ideas are worthy as a first-year teacher, but guess what? They are.)
- How will you be positive and travel to the unknown? (Education is full of change and the unknown. There is no way ever to be utterly prepared; stay positive.)
- How will you gain the gift of time daily, weekly, or yearly? (You will never finish every task—it just cannot be completed.)
- How will you visualize success for the day, week, and year? (Visualization works—take things at the moment and reflect.)

- What measures will be taken to travel to celebrations? How will this look inside the classroom, big/small, and daily/weekly/monthly? How will you celebrate yourself personally and healthfully?

STORY TIME

A young teacher wanted to be adored by her students. The mentor noticed after a student reported it; it was too late. One early morning, the teacher allowed the student to get in her purse, look at pictures of her boyfriend and family, and read love letters. Later, without permission, another student attempted to do the same thing. The teacher ran around the classroom, chasing the young man, trying to gain her purse back from the child. Finally, she retrieved her belongings from the student. Unfortunately, the relationship boundaries could not return to the correct state.

Chapter 5

Professionalism

Teachers are public figures in their communities. Their activities on and off the job are often scrutinized. Professionalism is an essential focus for a new educator. It is necessary to understand that everyone is watching behaviors at all times. Certain behaviors may send adverse inferences and be looked down upon by administrators, parents, and even students scathingly. The new educator needs to review the traits below and remember to put the best foot forward when traveling through their career.

It will take time and work, but the educator can master all of these traits:

- commitment
- confidence
- responsibility
- honesty
- ethics
- appearance
- dependability

When a teacher is professional in all areas, they carry themselves with the proper etiquette in a very positive manner. How will one communicate about the district, parents, and students? Time to critically reflect on actions. It is easy for some to become disconnected and feel permission to slip into improper behavior outside of the school day. Take special notice that places like restaurants, traveling, or social media can feed misbehavior.

Take heed and completely understand; administrators see and notice things one might not think they do. Posting on Instagram and Facebook is always entertaining until the wrong photo, post, or comment gets out. Be cautious of wearing one's spirit wear or any school logo in situations that can place things in a bad light. One way to look at it is not to post on social media situations that one would not want their grandmother to see. Please do not post it.

When socializing at school, try and keep personal matters to a minimum. Everyone wants to hear the good news, fun times, and family events, but it can easily become a distraction and take away from the job at hand. Keep in mind that teachers are here to do a job. Tiny ears and eyes are always listening and watching. Catch-up times will be available at lunch or after school.

Unfortunately, no one wants to wallow in an unfortunate series of events. It can start to become an easy distraction and take away from the job at hand. Most importantly, it will drag the teacher away from the positive circle. Try to lift others. Do not set a mission to make other teachers look bad. Do not enter the profession of education as an "us vs. them." Remembering we are all on the same team will continue to promote success for teachers and students. The students will be the winner in the end, and we will all celebrate the victories.

Be mindful at all times of your surroundings and understand your representation is influential. Showing up and acting like one who is genuinely invested in the school community will reflect professionalism.

Simply taking notes, asking quality questions, and listening during district meetings will reflect a professional manner. Body language is noticeable: sit up, look interested, and be engaged in every meeting. Show that one is ready to receive information and eager to learn and grow.

Problems and issues will arise in the school year with others; deescalate emotions before speaking. Do not regret words at the end of the day. Emails will overwhelm teachers from day one. Please choose a time to respond when one can think about a clear and positive response. If one is heated and this might happen, walk away. Do not send the initial email; you might feel the need to type and get emotions out. Advice will be to walk away, calm down, and revisit later. Be cautious of how the voice is perceived in an email.

Choose words and tone carefully so as not to hurt feelings or make matters worse. A good choice might be to allow the mentor or thinking partner to support and review before sending. Look like the leader that entered the building with those high hopes on day one. Everyone is watching; what will it look like for the educator to be professional?

Reflections:

- How will you acquire the look of professionalism in the first meeting?
- What will the plan for posting to social media look like for the teacher?
- How will you understand the cultural norms of the building?
- How will tone come across in voice, both face to face and in email?

STORY TIME

A new teacher arrived at the meeting early and set up the activity for the principal. She saw things that needed to be achieved and took the initiative, even though she could have made a phone call, grabbed coffee, or talked outside in the hallway with co-workers. The principal left the meeting discussing how the new teacher was heading to prominent places.

Chapter 6

Intentions and Best Practices for Learning

How will an educator sustain the positive circle and keep the best intentions while successful relationships and learning are occurring at all times? Once the connection is present, teachers will need knowledge of the content. In addition, new teachers often need more practice in the area of delivering the lessons.

    The students will need the teacher to be confident and know the content. They will need to feel the teachers' expertise, passion, and confidence. Practice will take time and work with an emphasis on setting each goal. The design of lessons, preparation, and understanding of data will be essential.

    The classroom will need to be very organized, with plenty of space for the flow and materials. Items will need to have a purpose and a place. If they don't, they are not needed. It will take a lot of reflection and revision for a first-year teacher to be successful. Implementation will not come easily, and each part of the process will need to be flexible and patient.

    It is the first year, and you will not have it all figured out. The content will need to be processed and taught in many different ways. It will be beneficial to discuss planning the lessons with teams of teachers, mentors, and coaches. Remember, there are professional developments to seek out if there is a lack of understanding in this area. Do not be afraid to speak up.

    One area that will be beneficial in the content area is understanding and implementing small-group instruction. The teaching days of whole-group instructions are gone. Unfortunately, this is not a comfortable area for most new teachers. Mostly since they were taught and modeled this way, they fall into the way they learned as a child.

    Take a risk and get to know the individualized prescription that each student needs. So much data is disaggregated in the classroom, and it will show a new teacher how to differentiate learning. It will take time to understand how to dive deep into the data and grow.

Find the different modalities in which students love to learn. Then, utilize an interest inventory at the beginning of school to understand each child better. Things will begin to fall into place; students will begin to fall in love with learning. The positive circle will begin to grow more extensive, and one will see authentic learning.

Reflections:

- How will you address setbacks and failures when teaching the content?
- What does it look like to set positive intentions with preparation and planning?
- How will the classroom continue to stay organized?
- What will your goal be for understanding data in the classroom?
- In what area do you need to feel confident?
- How does one utilize a voice when expressing difficulty?

"I can make a choice to let it define me, confine me, refine me, and outshine me, or I can choose to move forward and leave the issues behind me and choose growth and reflection."—Unknown

STORY TIME

A rookie practitioner pulled a small group together only to discover that a student placed in a high group was not reading at the correct level. It had been weeks later, and he suddenly realized the student had accommodations needed to obtain growth and that the specific needs had not been met. Adjustment to instruction occurred, and the student grew an entire grade level by the end of the year. Without the time and proper accommodations, the student would not have received proper instruction, and no growth would have occurred. It's important to know the student's abilities.

Chapter 7

Lesson Preparation

Developing and practicing lesson plans in advance is necessary to be prepared and confident. With a well-developed and rehearsed plan, students will see your conviction and credibility. They will feel a passion for the subject and gain confidence in their ability to learn.

Planning seems to be the most difficult for a first-year teacher. It is because it takes hard work, time, and critical thinking skills. Invest time, weekly, and monthly on planning and preparing lessons. Remember, if something does not work out correctly, then go back and try it again differently. If there is no plan, a new teacher will lack confidence and things will not go well. A new teacher cannot and should not walk into a classroom without a prepared agenda. It is not only necessary to plan a step-by-step lesson but also be familiar with the content. One example would be reading the book prior to teaching it.

Training and preparation have prepared one to become a professional educator. However, it will take mental strength, hard work, and time to plan lessons, especially if one is self-contained with many subject areas to teach.

Most districts have protocols to follow that make planning a lesson much more manageable. If it becomes a struggle, involve the mentor and learn the steps. Most districts have coaches that can support new teachers. Reach out and ask for help; people honestly will want to support you. Utilize your voice and speak up, and gain the support needed to be well planned. Invest in the time and create daily reminders to travel to the positive side, and the plan will be a success.

- What is the topic of the lesson?
- What is it that students need to learn?
- What will students do at the end of the lesson?
- What will the task of the lesson include?
- Are you using worksheets because it is easier than planning?
- What will the takeaway from the lesson include?

Occasionally, life will happen, and days will come when the teacher needs to be outside the classroom. It will be necessary and mandatory to stay prepared. Substitute plans will be required, so students do not lose learning time and ensure the substitute teacher feels supported and comfortable leading the class. The teacher will want everything ready for the substitute to be successful in his or her place. Remember, the positive circle is respectful at all times. It will be necessary to create this planning box early on in the school year. When you have a plan in every area, you can sigh a breath of relief.

Substitute Plan Checklist:

- Substitute folder or binder with detailed information.
- Binder is in clear view at all times.
- Class list of every period/seating chart for each period/class.
- Class rules and procedures/special needs/allergies, etc.
- List of students from each period who are leaders and can support if necessary.
- Phone list of administrative contacts/emergency numbers.
- A map of the school.
- Collection of books, articles with questions, or engaging activities (leave in the binder for emergency times when you cannot get to the school).
- Location in your room where you leave the emergency plans.
- Number and plan to notify a "work person" of where you have left the emergency plans.
- Understanding campus-specific procedures when requesting an absence.
- Contact your principal for permission.
- You are not alone; it is all about becoming a team.

Reflections:

- Does the lesson plan have a clear objective?
- How will it be measured and specific?
- How will you hook the learner at the beginning of the lesson?
- Do the students know the "why" prior to the lesson?
- Are the activities well- planned and prepared?
- Is there an opener and a closure to the lesson?
- Have you planned for the time of the lesson?
- How will you identify mastery of the lesson?
- Is the room organization ready for small groups, friendly, and organized?
- Is there a plan for technology, plugs, and chargers?
- Are you familiar with policies, room numbers, and phone numbers?

- What is the school plan for supplies? What will be community and individual?

STORY TIME

After a new teacher returned to school from being ill, a student came up and told her the sub was very nervous and jittery. The class thought it was odd when she gathered her purse on the way to P.E. "She took us to our specials class and just kept walking straight out the door. She never returned, and the principal taught the class for the rest of the day." Then, a few days later, a young man told the principal that they were so happy to see the return of their teacher. The moral of this story is always to be ready; you never know what the sub will bring to the table.

Chapter 8

New Mindset and Self-Care

Let us begin to paint a clear picture in this chapter about the correct mindset and self-care of an educator. The importance of a positive mindset should be practiced daily for many reasons. Studies show it increases a lifespan, induces better health, and creates a more positive impact on those around. It provides clear thinking, better moods, and better coping skills. Also, it allows a person to be more creative and calmer.

Some ways to become more positive are meditating, keeping a gratitude journal, spending time with positive people, enjoying hobbies, watching something funny, and creating morning and evening rituals. Oftentimes beginning breathing techniques can be helpful. Taking time to create self-talk and reframe the story one tells oneself can be beneficial.

New teachers need to learn a balance within their lifestyle. Understanding being good to oneself increases happiness and improves energy. With all the extras added in teaching, sometimes a pause will be necessary. Listen to the body and readjust expectations.

Teachers are in a new place right now, preparing to be genuinely ready for the first year of school. The checklist is continuing to be revisited, intense training is completed, and rooms are fully decorated.

Unfortunately, some educator programs do not seem to prepare the newest educator on self-care and keeping the balance of life. Somehow the best intentions and energy start to change around September. Many are finding that no money is left in their pockets. Feelings of excitement and exhaustion are occurring in the body and mind. Many are finding out that the preparation for students has been much harder than ever expected. The mindset that one must discipline, love, and teach high-level, tech-savvy kids is finally hitting home. The belief must remain clear to conquer the year with success and the mindset to bring it on! The profession is full of challenges, with decisions that one will not always be a part of but mandated to follow.

You will not need to stay hours at work and neglect home life even if you are single. Most people who enter the profession are achievement-oriented and can easily pour heart and soul into the craft. Quickly find a balance and schedule a time for self-care.

Suppose one develops a mindset where one works when it is work time, and one finds the balance needed to succeed. How will mental preparations begin to support how one spends their time and thoughts? One recommendation is to stop comparing oneself to others. If someone is staying long hours, do not let them guilt others into staying later than anticipated. Instead, invest in balance to get work done during working hours.

Be aware and understand that the list will grow longer and never quite become completed in education. It is just the reality of the career. The truth is that education is endless, and one can and will always be working on it.

Soon nutrition may become an area of concern for new teachers. It will be necessary to pay attention to the selection of food. Is one choosing healthy instead of junk food? It is effortless to grab a bag of candy or soda because one feels bad, which always seems to make one feel better at the moment. Sugar intake is not the fix. It will only make a body sluggish and tired.

Try to start the day with a good breakfast or at least an energizing smoothie of some sort. Some easy examples for meal prepping will be utilizing small storage containers, ready for lunches and dinners. Make a plan, get a menu, and keep a calendar with workout days.

Great recipes are available for excellent, healthy smoothies. Be conscientious of caffeine intake; too much coffee will send one over the edge during the day. A big crash will inevitably occur, and concentration can be lost.

Train the mind to make a conscious effort to grab veggies or fruit. Drinking water is difficult because most classrooms do not have a water fountain or bathroom. However, water is necessary for a clear mind and endless energy. Finding time to get the intake will find a cleanse and clarity for the mind. Vitamin C will become a best friend, allowing health to become the top priority. Children are counting on teachers to show up daily. One must remember to take daily care seriously.

Finding time to exercise is a must for all teachers, even just a few times a week. Intentionally block off time to at least get out and take a nice walk. A first-year teacher will be exhausted when arriving home. It will be necessary to plan out the exercise and hold oneself accountable. Sometimes having a workout buddy will help.

If the new teacher is without a hobby, quickly choose one; it will be necessary for keeping sanity. It will be necessary to remain active and create a healthy lifestyle. The new teacher will need to choose fun activities, so they remain consistent. Some fun examples might be martial arts, yoga, weightlifting, or a nice walk. Take time for a massage or spa day to treat yourself. Read a great book, journal thoughts, dance, or call a friend. Make yourself laugh or have a good cry; both are good escapes. Often blocking out all emails after six o'clock can be beneficial. Self-care is about doing something that makes one feel good emotionally, physically, or mentally.

Shoes can make or break a new teacher's day. What is one choosing to wear on the feet today? Corns, calluses, bunions, ingrown toenails, or plain sore feet can seriously ruin a great day. People throughout history have placed shoes on their feet that look fabulous and headed out the door expecting a great day of compliments, only hours later to find blisters are occurring, and soreness is creeping in. Sadly, the focus has turned only to the feeling in the feet.

Certain thoughts will begin entering the mind like this is it; one cannot continue on another moment. One may get stuck in a classroom overseeing children in the teaching profession, realizing there is no time for a break. Educators know that one cannot just take one's shoes off and run around the room. Plan and wear comfortable shoes to work. One recommendation is to bring two different pairs to school. Then, change mid-day into a different pair of shoes to remain in comfort. Finally, begin to gain that explicit understanding that, if the feet hurt, teachers are no good to themselves or anyone else.

Seek out the balance to continue a healthy and happy journey. Take the time to take a deep breath, meditate, and get plenty of sleep at night. It will support the teacher to remain in the right frame of mind to stay healthy. Sometimes even taking a moment in between classes to get some fresh air will provide energy.

In addition, starting each week with a healthy meal plan will ease and support the stress and prevent educators from embarking on the dark side—the dreaded bad eating guilt. Fight the urge to stress eat and make good choices. Put down the sugar; do not reach for the handful of candy. Teachers can do it; make significant decisions daily. Honor the need to maintain a healthy body, believe and stay strong, and stay healthy.

Unknowingly teachers may fall into a destructive pattern, making poor choices and neglecting their health. Be conscientious and do not beat yourself up when mistakes occur. Every day should reflect a new day for nutrition and health. Be mindful of self-talk; it is an enemy when it takes you outside the positive circle.

Some examples of healthy lunches for new teachers to pack are:

- salad in a jar containing lettuce, tomatoes, and favorite veggies
- nibbles for the day: pack nuts, veggies, carrots, apples, or granola bars
- cucumbers and hummus
- whole wheat tortilla with pizza sauce and cheese
- crackers, cream cheese, and bell peppers
- chicken salad with flax seed crackers
- turkey and cheese wrap

- meal prep a burrito bowl: ground beef, cheese, lettuce, tomatoes, onions, and sour cream
- leftover rotisserie chicken with a side of watermelon
- oatmeal and bananas
- whole wheat pasta with broccoli or asparagus

Reflections:

- What will your workout plan look like for the first week, month, and year of school?
- How can you be gentle with yourself daily?
- What will the food preparation look like for the first week, month, and year?
- How can you stay positive when you feel tired and terrible?
- How will you use your best efforts in not having an active lunch account in the cafeteria?
- What will your hobby be other than teaching?

STORY TIME

A new teacher remembered the first year started strong with eating well. Christmas time arrived, and she had gained ten unforeseen pounds, and realized she was lethargic and tired all the time. Heading back to school, she decided to throw away all the candy on her desk to help her make better choices. A boy turned to her and said, "You could come to my house tonight. I do not want to eat my vegetables anymore. I will gladly give them to you, because I love you."

Chapter 9

The Pessimist Syndrome

Suddenly there comes a time when one cannot seem to do anything correctly at school or in life. The meetings are coming more often, and time is minimal. Nevertheless, it will seem quite often that everyone wants a piece of time. The educational profession will be challenging; at some point, one will inevitably want to quit. The new educator ponders if they must say yes to everything and everyone. How can anyone be the best at everything?

The expectations are too high to conquer. The work is too hard, and the people do not care how it feels to be working nonstop in the district. There will be a day when the voice inside your head is saying things such as, "not a good teacher, wife, husband, parent," and the list of negatives go on and on. The criticism is seeping into one's thoughts hourly and daily.

Constant processing of information will be occurring at all times. It could quite possibly be that one is tired and needs rest. Seeking opportunities for mindfulness, not frustration, will be essential when these voices appear, and they will. Preserve how to value oneself daily, often remembering fear is illogical. Remember, so much of the job will get easier with hands-on experience and knowledge. Therefore, it will be crucial at times and essential to replace any negative thoughts with positive phrases such as everything one is doing is beneficial. The work is hard but worthy. It matters daily to kids.

Reflect and complete a reality check to see if one is really in a dire situation when thoughts are imploding in the brain. It quite honestly might be time to take a moment, close one's eyes, take a breath, reflect, and collect thoughts logically. Then, stop the negative thoughts and figure out how to make the changes needed for results. Do not allow things to get distorted and spiral out of control. The negative thoughts will show up often as fear, doubt, or mere anxiety.

Remember the new educator is embarking on the rewarding mission of getting to mold children into adults. It is the first year as a teacher; remember who the hero is at this job. Rethink the thoughts and shift the perspective. Begin to guide the imagery and keep the focus off distractions. Sometimes honestly, naming the actual problem can be pretty helpful. It is a long process, but educators must continue the ongoing mind, body, and spirit training. Furthermore, this will take ongoing practice.

The next tip is to continue to create daily reflection times. Look and reflect on all the good things happening. If one cannot find any, look to a mentor or coach for support. Honestly, take the time to listen and accept that one is more than the negative thoughts. Understand that one has entered the most valuable profession, educating children.

Take the time to check to see how body language looks and how one is positively carrying oneself. It can quite possibly be a huge step toward success. For example, when students look at a teacher's body language, it can show a lot. Standing up straight; walking with pride and confidence can help make a positive impression.

Students, staff, and administrators will need to believe that you are in the correct profession. It will draw in others, and everyone will want to hear the words out of your mouth. Become the magnetic energy that rubs off on others. Feeling powerful and positive can be accomplished if practiced often. What positive words will the new educator practice during the first week, month, and year of school?

Work on being an active listener in every situation. A few tips when struggling: close your mouth and listen to someone speaking. Look a person in the face and keep eye contact with them and hear what they have to say. Understand someone's perspective before beginning to judge what they are saying or doing.

Remember, research shows that relationships increase academic achievement. Therefore, the relationship with oneself will always continue to matter. Finally, celebrate the achievement; one has done good today, serving kids is the greatest gift, the path matters, and be a success today and every day.

Reflections:

- How can you remain in a space where you can get all the facts?
- How can you understand that something may be only a perspective, not reality?
- Where can you go to obtain more information about an issue?
- How can you not make rash decisions?
- How will you face criticism and what will the strengths look like?
- How will you meet failure?
- How will a plan be created to balance life as an educator?
- How will bringing students to the forefront daily and celebrating success support education?

STORY TIME

A new teacher began feeling the emotion of frustration. She was always arriving late to school. Unfortunately, this put her behind in starting her day positively. She understood that negative emotions were emerging in the tone she used with students. Communicating with a mentor teacher, they got to the bottom of the real issue and traveled to a solution. She came up with a plan to have her wake up earlier every morning. Owning the emotion and having a thinking partner, she was able to travel to a solution very quickly. Soon realizing beginning the day cheerful and not rushed, she was able to let the frustration go and remain positive.

Chapter 10

One, Two, Three: Evaluator and Me

It is time to feel safe in the culture of the school workplace where taking interpersonal risks are celebrated. It is not the place to ignore, reject, or ridicule. One of the hardest hurdles for a new teacher is being evaluated and feeling judged. If you are in the correct mindset, growth can be gained, instead of unnecessary stress. Prior to school starting, obtain a copy of your school district's evaluation system. Gather all district information related to it. Review your personal goals and set specific goals for the school year with your administrator.

Expectations will be set to collect data and evidence throughout the school year. Prepare a mindset to expect people traveling into your classroom for observations. Work and become comfortable with the open-door policy. Remember to keep good communication skills at all times with all coworkers. Do not listen to gossip, false stories, or accusations. New teachers are very naive about the practice of teaching and must remember to go to an accredited person for answers. Do not be afraid to ask tough questions.

Allow yourself time to grow as a new educator. It will help to develop the mindset that evaluators can and will offer advice in areas to help you improve. Having a growth belief system and adopting the mindset that you can succeed will set you up for success. Keep perspective that a new teacher is still in the growth process. Also, understand that you bring great things to the table.

For example, if a walkthrough is done in your classroom, and you are having an off day; your evaluation is not quite as successful as you would have liked it to be. Instead of jumping to conclusions that you let everyone down, take a deep breath and understand that everyone has a bad day. Teachers are humans—not robots.

Maintain open communication with the administrator about what happened and move back into the positive circle as quickly as possible. Negative self-talk can damage teachers; keep it out of the thought process. Instead, have a well-planned lesson, set goals, and communicate, and the process will be more straightforward.

It is vital to know that the educator will most likely not hit the exceeded mark in all areas in the evaluation process. It is acceptable to receive a low rating during the first year on the job. If this occurs, let this motivate you to continue to work and strive to get better. Set a mindset to be okay with the place and time of this moment. Striving for perfection is great, but it can lead to disappointment. One must strive for growth instead, and be open to all feedback.

We must be still and reflect on things slightly more. If we place ourselves in others' shoes, we can visualize a different perspective. We must try and visualize it and the meaning behind it. Educators must let go of always being right. We are on the same team at all times. We must listen to, understand, and not always reply with an answer.

Training yourself to commit to respectfully hearing what others have to say may take time and practice. Try allowing others to respond to a comment and have some good self-reflection time. A true understanding of what someone has to say may take more time. Try and allow yourself this time and then get back to them and discuss them. I believe as new teachers, we are always ready to hear the negative—try and start expecting positive words about your performance. Begin to really listen objectively to the administrators. Most of the time when hearing any negative criticism, you have already begun addressing it and are fully aware of the problem.

Remember to keep an open mind—it does no good to become defensive. Try again to really listen to the takeaway. Is it about daily practice? If so, do not take it so personally. Once one has reflected, think of the ways to continue to move forward. Remember, tomorrow is a new day.

Keep your administrator posted on new things you are experimenting with and growing with your practice. Utilize their advice and chunk out ways to improve. Most of all, keep growing. If you find yourself stressed out during the first phase of teaching, try and understand where it is coming from and find a go-to solution.

Place thought into how possibly the problem could be solved without alerting others. Is it possibly too early to panic and alert the authorities? It is easy to complain but you must reflect and sometimes make a personal change in order to grow.

Why is confidence so low? Answer: trust is missing. "Trust is confidence born of the character and competence of an individual or organization."[1]

Reflections:

- Is there an understanding of the learning target of the lesson?
- How is feedback from the administrator changing the practice?
- What are the goals for the lesson?
- What do you expect the outcome of this lesson to look like?
- How will you explain the process?
- Did you accomplish the goals?
- What could you have done differently?
- Is your management plan working or do you need to reflect and change?
- If and when things are not working, ask yourself *why*?

STORY TIME

An administrator reflects on a new teacher that had a scheduled observation in late October. Entering the classroom, the teacher told the administrator to come back another day. She replied that things were not going the way she wanted them to today. The administrator looked at the students, and they replied, she said if we were perfect, we could have an ice cream party on Friday. The novice teacher realized she needed to be more prepared and well planned. She learned to keep communication open with her administrator.

NOTE

1. Covey, Stephen M. R. "How the Best Leaders Build Trust." LeadershipNow. (2002). Accessed May 1, 2021. https://www.leadershipnow.com/CoveyOnTrust.html.

Chapter 11

Life outside of School

New educators must remain in the positive circle, and others will begin to gravitate. Life will occur outside of education, and school hours do not accommodate it. Soon, the new teacher will realize that they may not even be able to go to the post office or the bank during the first year of teaching because of irregular hours. It takes an effort to manage time and figure out how to balance home and school. It might take creative ways, but a school and home balance can emerge. Ask for assistance with a plan if necessary.

Wrap your head around what your plan will be when these things arise. You are now responsible for the lives of children. You have different priorities now because the children need a quality teacher daily. How will your balance look? Throughout the school year, we have to revisit our balance. It is easy to pull away and only focus on one area in life. However, without balance, students and the new teacher will begin to suffer.

Career, personal, physical, family, mental, spiritual, and financial priorities can become overwhelming. New teachers keeping the balance will remain prosperous and healthy. Education is a lifestyle commitment; sometimes it might feel selfish, but one must take care of their health. Finding the acceptance and respect of all parties will allow for connectedness. Reference and redirect the balance as one travels through one's positive circle. You will see listed below life encounters that could occur during your first year.

If one encounters a lack of balance, how will the choice to react come across? What will the attitude look like in the classroom? How can one keep the balance and be the success one needs to be? Finding when new educators begin teaching, the outside world still revolves daily. One must prioritize the outside world. Many things will need to be accounted for in the personal life. It is okay to take one afternoon and go get things done. Stop with the guilt—guard the self-talk.

One of the biggest problems with teachers is tardiness to school. You must be on time—students wait for no one. Compare it to a flight attendant or pilot; if you're late you are keeping hundreds of people from departing. Do whatever it takes to be on time. When things do come up, and they will, communicate and have a good team to cover your back.

Remember, do not take advantage of people; this will keep things positive. Stay in the positive circle and be the light—you can do this; it is your calling. Pointed out are conditions that may arise as a first-year teacher. Be aware of triggers and thoughts prior to unexpected situations occurring.

Checklist for Unexpected Situations:

- Time Management: How can you possibly fit everything into the day, week, and month? Remember to create a balance and plan.
- Money Management: How can you possibly make it until payday? Remember to create a budget and plan.
- Relationship Problems: How can you possibly teach with everything going on at home? Remember, once at school, place everything out of the head except teaching.
- Balance: How can you possibly do everything that everyone needs one to do? Remember, a new teacher cannot take on extra the first year.
- Insecurities in relationships? How can you gain the approval of people in the district? Remember to start with yourself and be respectful of others.
- Death of a loved one: How will you allow yourself to grieve yet continue to focus on the students? Remember, sometimes students will give you the support and keep the mind busy and begin to heal.

Note: Remember that unexpected events will happen in one's life. Begin to understand and accept that it can and will often happen in life. Create learning opportunities along the way and be reminded that one can always speak with someone they trust about issues. Take heed to guard thoughts and go to the positive circle. Reflect on the problem and travel to the solution. See problems and mistakes as a growing opportunity, keep a sense of resilience, and travel to balance as often as possible.

Reflections:

- How will you stop comparing yourself to others and at all times keep a positive growth mindset?
- What will open communication look like with administrators?
- How can you train your mind to balance daily items?
- What area will you need to focus the most on this week?
- How will you notice if an area needs more attention?
- Who will you seek out for support?
- What will the plan be for unexpected issues?
- Who is you first contact person?
- What is the plan for arriving on time?

STORY TIME

A new teacher lost a loved one during the first year of teaching. She had to deal with many outside stressful personal responsibilities. Unfortunately, this meant time away from her students. Suddenly, after the grief had settled, she realized the school family was there to support her. Somedays, tears flooded, and a teammate would take her class while she composed herself. She received the much necessary support and love needed to continue down a successful path. The lesson learned was that relationships truly matter in the education world. Sometimes they are the only things that may get a person through the difficult times.

Chapter 12

New Teacher Growth in the First Year

Begin to gain an understanding that growing in a teaching craft will never cease. No one will ever arrive in a place where they are experts on everything. Education is such a unique profession that it is ever-changing. A new teacher will reflect on how to continue to grow. One might wonder why this is important the first year when survival is all that is on the mind.

The new educator must decide the area in which they want to grow and improve in the first year. After choosing this area, one must be ready for coaching. New teachers often feel like they are living in a bubble. So many times, these young educators place this upon themselves. Perception can take on many different looks throughout the first year. It takes reaching out and gaining feedback to grow. Through the correct mindset, support, and resources, confidence will build, and new educators will thrive, not just survive.

Teachers can gain the mindset to always be growing in the craft. One manner in which to begin to grow in their craft is by utilizing professional learning communities as well as learning walks. The community improves the skill and knowledge of educators. It provides opportunities for collaboration and professional dialogue. Oftentimes, it allows teachers to question, evaluate, and improve knowledge.

A learning walk is when a colleague visits another classroom to view instruction. It is nice to even take a few minutes to look at the flow of the classroom. Usually, leadership is very happy to assist in scheduling these opportunities. Time is a shortage as a new teacher but if you will find time to observe other teachers' instruction you can continue to grow.

There are many aspects of the profession you can observe and learn from others. It is amazing what you can take away in a brief ten-minute timeframe. Even the greatest educator can learn from others in their practice. The biggest thing is to continue to grow.

At the beginning of the year, professional development can seem overwhelming. One manner in which districts can support new teachers is by providing actual scenarios instead of lecturing through the topic. New teachers need actual management training due to the fact that this is not always provided at the college level. Opportunities may be provided for new teachers to reenact difficult situations and create action plans.

As I have stated earlier, creating an academy for these teachers and meeting at least once a month will provide the support system needed for the "buy-in" to retain teachers. An outline for this type of academy will be provided in this book. New teachers will need to be open to attending these academies or meetings.

We must look at professional development prior to school as the final dress rehearsal. Allow time for developing routines and procedures with practice. Administrators can support with feedback and by showing a bit of a personal side prior to school beginning. It is a time for districts to begin to reflect and create a strategic plan of action alongside new educators.

It is imperative to remember that the new teacher is the greatest asset to the district and the classroom. You are responsible for facilitating your students' engagement, growth, and well-being. It is the biggest responsibility ever given to any human. And, in case you don't invest in the asset—the new teacher—the students will be impacted greatly in negative ways.

Stay in the positive circle and be those amazing educators who are hungry to learn and grow in practice. Enter the field with a growth mindset, ready to master education. In the teaching career, if one stops growing, one will need to find a new profession. It is not fair to children. If one is not happy, reanalyze the profession. Remember, it will not be easy, but it is worth it. The children count on the teacher daily. It is a considerable weight to carry, and it must be at the forefront of minds at all times. So, one has just finished college, and yes, one still needs to grow.

Districts must keep their mindset on creating a school culture of lifelong learners. Frequently, our new teachers are afraid to show vulnerability. It is okay not to know everything the first year. Teachers are generally coming from a background of mainly learning theory. Now teachers will be shifting to the "doing" aspect. It is essential to gain the support necessary and learn new approaches along the way. What style works for one educator might not work best for others.

The new teacher must realize that everything takes practice. It is essential to understand that teachers must practice something at least three times to start to get into a routine. The new teacher needs to understand what practice can be taken for the quickest growth. Often new teachers do not put in the practice, either because of time or confusion. Remember, motivation, self-reflection, and much inspiration will bring confidence to a new teacher. Put in the time and practice for proper growth.

We must support the new teacher by understanding the practice of a routine and putting these steps into action will gain improvement. It will take all district employees to support. It is evident that placing a first-year teacher on an island is placing our students at a considerable disadvantage and possibly a place where recovery cannot happen.

New teachers must be open to supporting and coaching in education. The support will allow risk and improvement to be immediate. We must look at teacher retention as a matter of urgency. The more quickly a teacher masters relationship skills (the most important skill of teaching), the more quickly students will learn. If you keep relationships and student achievement at the forefront, you will become the educator, you were meant to be.

Understanding how and developing a reflective practice takes time. This book has set reflection topics for each chapter, but one must incorporate this practice into daily life. Some examples of reflection might be a sticky note, journal entry, or video. Set an intention to reflect on practice and record your outcomes. It is important to choose a way to become reflective and then stick to it. Along with a great place to house thoughts, it will also be a great place to see trends in education. Believe and carry the mindset that this kind of reflection allows us to stay positive when we see ourselves slipping into a dark education hole.

Teaching trends can sometimes be very overwhelming when maneuvering through the educational world. The pendulum swings and educators must be flexible when it moves quickly. Setting goals will be a path to success, no matter how big or small. One needs to see it to work toward it. One may not always meet the goal, but learning will occur along the way.

Checklist:

- What is keeping you from moving forward in the daily teaching practice?
- What support do you need to move forward and who needs this support at the campus level or district level?
- How will you ask for support appropriately?
- What action will you take once the support is given?
- How will you feel having those uncomfortable conversations?
- What routines for instruction have been implemented and do you need to adjust practices?
- What classes are you enrolled in to continue growth?
- Why are you doing certain strategies, and are they successful?
- Are you allowing opportunities for students to show what they know?

Reflections:

- What district seminar or book study are you participating in for the year?
- What are the measures of success?
- How is curriculum planning and data assessment supporting your growth?
- How will you make a plan and reach out for modeling and coaching?
- How are you reflecting on practices at this point in the year?

STORY TIME

A new educator began to struggle with teaching the content. Being extremely shy, she did not want to bother anyone. The mentor teacher noticed the struggle. She supported and helped her discuss with the principal a class that offered support in the specific content. The educator attended, and she reframed her mindset. After this, the new teacher joined a book study and showed much progress as she finished her first year. Her lesson was to utilize one's voice early if a teacher begins to struggle. District personnel truly want teachers to be successful.

Chapter 13

Teacher Retention

Limitless studies specify that teachers are the greatest significant influence on any student's schooling. So why can't we keep good teachers? Retention of teachers was found to be related to three broad themes:

- Teachers' strong interpersonal relationships and community ties in rural communities.
- School factors include a positive school environment, contact between teachers and administrators, interpersonal relationships with students, and flexibility.
- Professional factors such as opportunities to teach intellectually stimulating subjects, the ability to connect topics to rural life, professional development opportunities, and a sense of job satisfaction and job security.[1]

Teacher retention is the buzzword around our nation today. However, administrators question why we cannot "keep" high-level educators in our schools or even in the profession. Many very educated people state it is because the salary is not high enough. Some state it is because the workload is too heavy. Others tend to believe it is quite frankly because kids are more demanding these days. The fact is that 40 to 50 percent of teachers are leaving the profession within the first five years.

Many schools are struggling to close the achievement gap because they never close the quality gap. They are constantly rebuilding their staff from year to year. It may be the first year of delivering instruction, but it is the students' only year to learn the content needed for success. We must strive to be effective in every way possible.

In order to keep newly excited teachers in the profession, teacher investment must be an integral part. Established positive relationships must start with those entering the field. It takes work and understanding to invest in these areas. A positive attitude and relationships are the key to the rise in education and student achievement. Positivity comes from both the brain and the heart. People struggle with what being positive and relational looks like and how to be successful in both areas.

Creating a clear pathway to support, develop, and build first-year teachers' skills will increase student achievement and teacher retention. In addition, creating many opportunities for growth and reflection along the way will impact the growth cycle.

But first, we must understand what the goal is. How do we get there? What is the district's plan, school's plan, and our plan? Generally speaking, it consists of these elements:

- Increase a student's love of learning daily
- Provide feedback when needed
- Decrease teacher turnover rate
- Invest in new teachers
- Increase new teacher effectiveness
- Increase teacher job satisfaction
- Provide strategic support and develop stronger relationships with teachers
- Grow teacher leaders
- Articulate and create investment in the district goal
- Make time to reflect
- Focus on building relationships
- Lean on mentors
- Expect to fail, understanding that improvement will occur
- Surround oneself with positive colleagues

Reflections:

- How will the pathway of support be organized in the start of the school year?
- What is the district plan to grow teachers?
- What will the mentor role be in supporting throughout the school year?
- Are the positive feedback options created to show this kind of investment?

STORY TIME

Midyear, a new educator realized the principal was leaving for a promotion outside the district. The teachers had built a relationship and were worried about what the future might hold. The evening after the announcement, the literacy coach stayed well into the evening, answering questions and settling the minds of those worried. Due to the support, it was the lowest turnover rate the district had ever had. The lesson learned was to invest time, and that communication matters to teachers.

NOTE

1. Goodpaster, Kasey P., Omolola A. Adedokun, and Gabriela C. Weaver. "Teachers' Perceptions of Rural Stem Teaching: Implications for Rural Teacher Retention." *The Rural Educator* 33, no. 3 (2018): 9–22. https://doi.org/10.35608/ruraled.v33i3.408.

Chapter 14

Administrator: Friend or Foe?

A good leader will be an asset to the educational system. It is crucial that the leader remains consistent with what they say and keeps credibility at the forefront of decisions. It will begin to set things in motion from day one. In high-needs districts, teacher retention is crucial. The chaos and lack of stability in students' home life deserve teachers who are there for the long haul. Unfortunately, research indicates that most new teachers will leave school because of a lack of support, poor professional development, and feeling like they are not heard or valued. Placing a new teacher in a classroom without support is like placing them in a cockpit as a pilot without the hours.

New teachers need a school climate where they feel a constant sense of success in the growing process. Respect by all is the key to this kind of success in the teaching profession. New teachers to the profession will hear one's words, but they also feel an attitude. New teachers are highly needy and must have that constant connection.

It will be necessary to form a team to support the administrators because they cannot do this alone due to time constraints. It is crucial in creating an understanding when interviewing, especially, for low socioeconomic schools. Teachers need to understand the job they are entering, and that support is available at all times.

The belief that kids cannot learn must become a view of the past and become abolished. Even though cultures can be different, these students are very capable of learning. Administrators must set the school climate with a commitment to all staff to retain our teachers and raise student achievement in all areas. Allowing new teachers to have a voice and feel empowered is very important in the first year. Do not perpetuate laziness; preserve something that one values.

The administrators are driven daily by mandates and duties. One main priority must encompass new teachers. Administrators sit in a lonely position in which one rarely receives gratitude. The weight lies heavily on the administration's shoulders. If we view our teachers as partners and keep the communication line open, we can be successful. New teachers need to hear positives almost daily from administrators.

They come to us with high expectations of themselves already. The daily grind makes it nearly impossible to meet all expectations they will put on themselves and administrators. Be cautious of gravitating toward the same teachers. Talk and reach out to all, not just the popular, outgoing ones. Keep oneself grounded and do not listen to gossip. Notice the good things.

The little things can mean an abundance. Administrators can send a daily email that has an inspirational quote or a positive note to teachers. They can walk around the building shaking hands and saying, "Good morning." We must check on new teachers and diminish fear daily. Sometimes it is just the little things. Entering conversations with empathy and listening to hear and sometimes not respond can be instrumental in conversations. Work to remain present, purposeful, and intentional in daily matters. Sometimes just an acknowledgment of the feelings of being overwhelmed and helping a new teacher prioritize can go a long way.

We must show that we value teachers even though the workload keeps growing. It is a fine line in trying to be a friend to new teachers. Administrators will inevitably gravitate to specific teachers. Sometimes they gravitate to the outspoken or popular teachers, but one must remember to remain in the professional area. Once the new teacher crosses over to eating lunch out, visiting homes, or just hanging out, it will be too late to coach them and see changes without hurt feelings.

All parties involved need to learn to let go of negative expectations. Keep the mindset to start over fresh daily. One of the most important virtues is integrity as an administrator. Actions speak very loudly to new teachers joining this wonderful profession.

Life will get busy and challenging. We are only human, but we must always keep our integrity at the forefront of our lives. We need to continue to travel in our positive circle even if others are not entirely on board yet. The number one factor that the administration must consider is how one will provide emotional support to new teachers. It is imperative not to group new teachers with seasoned teachers.

Think if at all times this meeting is crucial. Does an administrator genuinely need extra coverage for a specific duty? Is the training essential to the new educator? Can we be utilizing them to pour into their practice instead? Unless it is necessary, please do not ask them to do it.

Be cautious of grouping teachers together and calling out negative items in a staff meeting. A strategically compliant teacher will genuinely believe that they are the teachers described and remember to travel to the individual and differentiate the discussions.

Check to make sure the new teacher is not overwhelmed with unnecessary emails. It is easy not to realize the amount of communication that may be traveling to a new teacher. Be alert to sending after-hour emails to new teachers. They are overwhelmed and exhausted and most likely will take everything way too personally.

Consider making a separate professional learning time during the week to meet with this particular group of educators. They need the extra time and support and will share more if differentiated. These educators need administrators on their side; do not let them down. True leaders inspire rookie teachers daily by persuading them to be the best they can be in a job that is difficult.

Stay in the positive circle and make a daily difference; it will impact student achievement. The primary purpose of instructional leadership is not to continually evaluate everything. Instead, try and support and develop the new teacher and, most of all, overcommunicate. We must focus on specifics and take action.

Our goal should be to coach these new teachers until mastery emerges. Daily feedback that involves the teacher taking ownership is necessary. We must take one skill at a time and build upon the previous ones to not overwhelm and burn them out of this profession. Asking new teachers questions will provide the time to reflect and understand the new practice. One does not know until one has reflected on or viewed someone else in the profession.

When discussing students, make sure one has facts and data to back it up. New teachers love to go off of a feeling or gut reaction. It is much better to look at student work, data, or a video for the best understanding. The need to support teachers' acquisition of new knowledge and expertise is vital. Administrators must understand how to support the new knowledge and expand on the expertise of our new educators. Collaborate with them on instructional design as well as expand on their new ideas while providing feedback.

Invest in professional learning to support the new educator. Real-time feedback can be very beneficial. Sometimes as an administrator, one is apprehensive about giving new educators leadership capacity. How can we allow those that are ready to move forward quickly?

Administrators need to understand ways to explain the new initiatives in bite-sized chunks, so new teachers are not overwhelmed. Sometimes administrators will find that when they discuss a problem, the new teacher will lack motivation or energy. In conversations, it can be stressed to the new teachers to seek out a solution.

Remember, this will take practice and time. Soon it will become a habit, which will benefit the administrator with less time spent on meaningless issues. There is a great need to provide the resources necessary to build these individualized successes. Ask the questions, and give support and praise. Yes, I said praise! Somehow, we seem to forget this component when we begin to lead others. Take time to write a note, call the classroom, give those shout-outs. Then, invest and watch what happens. Individuals like to be successful!

We want these new educators to stay on our mission and in our profession, and most of all, in the district that hired them. However, the administrator must remember that these novice eyes are watching and doing their best to learn at all times. Everyone enters this service industry wanting to be the very best and to serve kids. If the new educator does not value the complexity of teaching or administrational decisions, they may find the education system overwhelming as problems occur. Understanding the diverse needs of oneself will be able to, allow for changes to transpire naturally in professional learning.

Administrators must be cautious and watchful for high absenteeism rates, issues with fatigue, changes in behavior, or physical appearance. If a teacher begins secluding themselves and being less social, someone needs to intervene with action steps. Sometimes it just takes an ear to listen for a few moments for the new educator to feel validated. The goal is to retain, new educators and grow in the educational profession. Most importantly in the district, they are hired.

First, however, the administrator must remember that these novice eyes are watching to see what the next move will be from the administrators and how to handle different situations. Districts need to provide a focus for professional development on mental health and self-care strategies to equip teachers with ideas and things to be aware of and note. This year will be heavy and unique. A special process that new teachers cannot predict. We must be ready for the need to provide success. An induction program can support a district with retention. The goal is always to decrease teacher turnover.

Districts can quite possibly arrive at increasing the capacity of teachers with extra support. Our primary plan and investment are for all students to receive the best instruction possible at all times. Districts will need to make a concerted effort to hire individuals we believe will be outstanding teachers for our students. By providing an effective induction and mentoring program, success will be imminent. One example might be to give specific ideas or scenarios and start with answering questions new teachers may have. Leaders may share their first-year teaching experience.

The new teacher must understand that every seasoned teacher and leader once was a new teacher. Show the side of one that walked in the trenches. Never lose sight of the boots on the ground. Noted below is a way to gain a connection with teachers. In addition, principals or school leaders can open up with a roundtable that includes these questions. Allowing new educators a chance to see the leaders more clearly makes them seen as a person. It creates a sense of connectedness early on in the school year. It will support new teachers to hear the answers to these questions early on in the school year.

Make a priority to set them up or succeed. Stick to the vision for districts to secure the resources necessary to expand the teacher's belief in themselves. One must increase the level of support as the year progresses. Therefore, the new teacher academies should be designed and carried out intentionally for support during the first few years.

In the early stages of developing the academies, the topics will need to be created, and roles will be assigned:

1. Decide who will be leading the academy and providing support.
2. Utilize the energetic leaders who are willing to pour into the craft.
3. Allow them to recognize the need to support others.

It will be necessary to have trustworthy leaders. Frequently, districts find mentors helpful while attending the academy for support. Oftentimes new teachers will be sharing things and showing a vulnerable side. Choose wisely not to diminish the trust, and it will be a time for the cheerleaders to support and replenish spirits. The positive circle of leaders will spread throughout the district if received and chosen carefully. A comfort zone is a beautiful place, but nothing ever grows there. Positive work must be done daily.

Some monthly topics for administrators to plan professional development are shown in the following list.

ADMINISTRATOR PRESENTATION TOPICS

- You matter: Why teacher attendance is crucial
- Goal setting
- Get to know you (cheers, fears, tears, and tough conversations)
- Classroom management
- Parent communication
- Data to know and share
- Differentiation techniques
- Why content matters
- Fresh start: Why relationships matter
- Evaluation information
- Data analysis

Reflections:

- How will you choose to become a role model?
- How will daily check-ins look for new teachers?
- How will you not get caught up in the agenda and see the new teachers?
- Explain what characteristics you think most successful teachers own.
- What are the expectations for your teachers? (be very specific)
- Teachers will often discuss the support they are receiving in the district. What does this look like for you as a principal/leader?
- What's a story of yours that you do not get to tell often enough?
- What advice can you give on how to avoid "new teacher" burnout?

STORY TIME

An educator reflected on the time invested in learning at the academy. The initial goal was to learn more content knowledge, but along the way, special lifelong bonds were formed and remain today. Emotionally, he stated, it was the location where he met his wife. He reflected and thanked the new teacher academy for becoming more successful in classroom practices and making the connections needed to form those unique bonds.

Chapter 15

Roll Out and Monitor

The roll out and monitoring of procedures will be an ongoing practice throughout the school year for the new educator. Many days it will seem like students have forgotten everything. Procedures and routines will take the new educator's time and patience. It will be imperative to travel back to understanding and the zone of practice time.

Ensure that there has been an established common language in which the learners feel empowered. If an individual is struggling, maybe the procedure is not understood or is too rigid; take time to reflect. Sometimes traveling back to the success criterion the class made together will help—telling the community that the rules were ones they created, not the individual. Often revisiting together can create an understanding of the meaning and a sense of urgency.

In the classroom, the morning meeting area is a powerful location. One suggestion is to have a small squishy ball that one could throw, and students could tell something that is on their minds. Sometimes it may be good, bad, or indifferent. Creating a safe classroom community that can listen with respect and without judgment will create accomplishments.

The new teacher will need to frequently revise routines and focus on areas that need more detail or are not meeting standards. Nevertheless, one cannot stress enough: *practice—do it again*. Have the students do the routine again if not done correctly. Do not move forward; stay true to one's accountability component. Teachers need to understand teacher radar. New teachers must see all students and know when they are off task.

The profession of teaching requires much energy at all times. One's eyes must see the entire room at all times. Many call this the *teacher with-it-ness,* otherwise known as teacher radar. It is a mandatory skill to be successful. New educators must create eyes in the back of the head that see everything.

The educator will create a glance-over for off-task behavior at all times. They need to set the atmosphere of looking and moving around often. It will be necessary to keep students guessing where one's location might be at all times. Begin early in your career, creating energy in the classroom. Kids become bored very quickly, and honestly, so do adults.

The pace needs to keep moving at a good speed. One will find that moving among desks and around the room's perimeter will deescalate the off-task behavior. Circulating the room will allow the teacher to monitor off-task behavior and allow student work to get noticed. It is easy to sit or stand by the student speaking, but the teacher must move away and observe all students.

Monitor and see everyone and become involved in the situations that are occurring. Make it fun, keep them guessing what one is about to do, and keep them positive and on task. If the off-task conversation begins, check out what it is and then pause it and reengage. In the past, educators would sit at a desk and remain motionless. Quite honestly, a new teacher does not even need a desk. It will just gain clutter and become a perch for negativity.

Remember, one may need to stop, get everyone back on track, and retune. Do not let the energy get sucked out of the room. Be creative, and always remember who the adult in charge is. Some ideas to reestablish clear expectations might be traveling back to the meeting area. Revisit what is working and what is not.

Always remember to celebrate first, then fix. If something is not working, do not continue it. Change things for success. Remember to begin to change things for success. The class will inevitably veer off track periodically. Sometimes students will set a purpose to derail a lesson. Be aware, and be ready. Regain the professional stance and give a clear expectation of what the purpose of the activity might be. The new teacher will then pick back up with a positive tone and energy.

Why would one continue with the lesson when no one is listening? Year after year, one will see a classroom where students who work together to learn and support each other become successful. If we show the students the importance of practice, goal setting, and success, we are limitless in this career. Remember the mission, and the new educator is here to reach a distinction. Stay in the positive circle. Reach for the stars daily.

First-year teachers need practice and an understanding that it is part of on-the-job training. Many days of training will continue to show classroom behaviors beginning to diminish, and remember to promote student discourse and allow built-in time to give immediate feedback successfully. The teacher often needs to give the students a clear picture of the day or lesson. Students frequently want to know the *why* of the lesson and explaining your reasoning for the lesson can allow students to become more receptive.

In college-level work, one became familiar with the strategy called "framing" the lesson because it includes parts at the beginning and the end of the lesson. In the beginning, the teacher states the daily learning objective(s) in concrete, student-friendly language to communicate a clear focus for the day's class. Utilizing "student-friendly" language to write the objective allows students to understand in kid language. If students do not understand the direction needed to attain achievement, a shutdown will occur.

Posting the objective and discussing it will allow students to see and visualize the learning. They are allowing students to reflect along the learning journey. It will be necessary for the new teacher to complete the objective in one lesson or class. In the end, there may be a closing question, product, or task.

It will allow the teacher to see what students accomplished daily and support them further if necessary. The task will show that the student has gained understanding. If not, the teacher will be able to reteach in a manner that will be of mastery.

Reflections:

- How have you cultivated a positive relationship with each student?
- How was the rollout planned for procedures?
- How are the routines monitored for success?
- Are you focusing solely on what you are doing in the front of the classroom or on the work that is actually on top of the student's desk?
- How will you practice the professional stance and positive tone?

STORY TIME

A classroom teacher saw a student acting up in the hallway. At the time, she stated, "You go to the back of the line." The student did not listen; the teacher then said, "Go to the back of the line, or none of us will be eating lunch." Suddenly, she realized she would lose either way. If the student did not go to the back of the line, she could not deny lunch to every student and she would lose respect. The lesson was learned that caution must occur in what we say with consistency. Do not say what you do not mean; all credibility will be lost.

The best way to ensure success is never to lose energy because things are not working as fast as you want them to. New educators must continue to build student self-confidence, remembering the targeted audience.

Chapter 16

Management

These are the most common statements from new teachers within the first year of education:

- How can I keep my classroom climate respectful of success and positive at all times?
- Help! My classroom is out of control . . .
- You do not understand—this group of kids is just different!
- I can't stop crying every day!
- I am so overwhelmed; this may be my last day!
- I can't do this anymore.
- Something is wrong with this curriculum.
- There is not enough time to teach.
- I am leaving this school for an easier school.
- No one here at this school understands me.
- I have never seen kids like this before
- I do not get any support!
- No one understands!
- Teaching is so difficult!

Emotional depletion is like a slow crack in the foundation of education. So often, educators are quitting because it is not what they pictured it to be. Kids can and often will be difficult. Remember to frame your mindset from the beginning; these are great kids. Unfortunately, some just come with baggage.

Frequently, new teachers are disheartened due to students not getting the consequences expected. It becomes even more evident when working with challenging students. Teachers will need extra support through these challenging times. Utilize the mentors and administrators to reach out and gain support and ask uncomfortable questions.

Remember, in order for someone to accept support, the other person must believe the correct intentions are at the forefront of the support. No one wants to feel or believe they are incompetent in trying to be successful in reaching their goal.

Typical classroom management is anything but typical as a first-year teacher. In college, many have studied theory and gained valuable information. Learning can transfer once the new teacher takes time to practice and gain feedback in a safe setting. The goal is to carry this practice effectively to the classroom. Let us begin to think harder and more innovatively on reflection about our practice.

Embrace flexibility to adjust to difficult situations in our first year. Overcome our doubts and fears, letting go of those things that are not serving us well in our daily lives. Utilize the knowledge to overcome problems as they occur.

In the next chapters, examples of difficult behavioral scenarios will be practiced. It will show the evidence of how relationships are the key to success. One of the biggest struggles that can break a new teacher is classroom management. Once the new teacher finds success in this area, they will become truly amazing at their craft. Often new educators are finding students enter the room with a lack of respect. Certain students may not give you eye contact; some may even fall asleep in class.

Often new teachers walk into situations that may be tougher than most. One example might be that school is already in session and a class is established. Trainings may not have prepared an individual how to handle these situations. Often times new teachers will turn into a role model that is not as kind due to fear.

Quite possibly, turning to the route of being a dictator may occur. Students are fearful of making the wrong move or saying the wrong thing in this kind of classroom. New educators must remember habits of success must be created, modeled, and taught. Many times, educators forget the modeling phase of the expectations. It is necessary to show students exactly what is expected of them in every situation. For example, when a student is asked to pay attention, a teacher must explain what that means to the student.

Often short-term compliance can occur for the teacher if they live in the land of discipline through consequence, but one will not gain overall classroom culture and self-discipline. The more one uses it, the less effective it becomes effective.

The most excellent teachers operate with influence and engagement to build positive classroom culture. Shift the perspective so that the new educator moves away from the negative characteristics such as yelling, condescending attitude, and just plain ignoring.

Navigate quickly to a culture of setting examples and respecting all the students at all times. In setting the expectations of the classroom, remember that everyone matters in the room. Daily consistency will be imperative. If not, stay true to the word; students will discredit the teacher, and the student will never perform academically. Remember back in the early chapters, getting to know the student will gain an understanding of the behavior.

Make the connection, find the interest, and, although sometimes difficult, look for something to love. Be consistent in the "what to do" expectation. Remember always to assume the best in students. Make it a point to assume the reason for non-compliance is a lack of clarity.

Example:
I will now model for you the correct behavior for sitting in a small group.

1. Track with eyes as the teacher will model.
2. Sit up straight with hands folded in your lap, eyes on the teacher.
3. Voices off.
4. Push chair back. Good. Now stand up. Model back the correct behavior.
5. Repeat as needed.

With classroom procedures one must place ownership on students. One way for students to continue the ownership process is to create a class book, PowerPoint, brochure, or illustrate procedures. Students should be in charge and own the responsibility at all times.

In the scenarios below, one will closely look at ideas and specific examples to implement into practice. It is imperative to have the first week well planned and overprepared. Think about bathroom procedures, hallway procedures, and supplies. The most minor thing can set a class into a tailspin. Stay calm and positive at all times.

Let students and parents know *the real teacher*. Think early on about what you would like to share to bridge the relationship. Do not use a sarcastic or abrasive tone. You will discredit yourself quickly and not be able to recover. Allow students time for movement. Please do not take away recess, P.E., or any other times when they can be active. Children need movement and change. According to research, adding physical activity to the classroom results in more focus. If kids see they can push manners to push the buttons, it will invite chaos.

Educators must find those unique talents in each child and celebrate them, not punish them. The educator must see success instead of the constant trouble. No one wants students to end up in jail or on the streets. Again, every child has that unique talent. One needs to think before sending a child to the office. It makes a teacher lose credibility early on in the year.

Two areas that will deserve a trip to the office would be safety and health. Be cautious and remain calm, knowing one can handle the situation and remembering who the adult is in the situation. A proper understanding is that rules must not be created too rigid. Some students will make it a mission to attempt and try to break them from the start. Rules should not be punitive, one example turning to a classmate to borrow a pencil. The new educator needs to focus on creating a safe and organized structured environment. Student achievement should exist and be practiced again at all times.

The following chapters will show evidence of actual management scenarios in which relationship has supported the forming of the key to success. New teachers must realize that if they master just one thing the first year, it must be classroom management. The following statement will blow one's mind! Kids are the same, whatever school district they may travel to in their careers. They want to be cared for, feel consistent expectations, and gain excitement about learning.

Stay in your positive circle. Does it really help to raise your voice and get flustered? The honest answer is no; you will lose all respect. You can choose to beat them down or empower them. The focus must be on a culture of a class community at all times and it must remain consistent. New teachers travel back to remember that everything revolves around the safety of your classroom. Keeping students safe at all times is the most crucial aspect of management. It is important to find one thing you love about each child. It may be difficult at first, but it is necessary, so find it—the quicker the better.

A new teacher must find a system of rules and a way to celebrate each day. I would recommend not to fall into what may have been modeled by your childhood teacher. Most of the management techniques from the "old school" days will not work. The days are gone of the highly strict classroom with a paddle hanging by the door.

Students want to feel a sense of belonging and part of the rule process. Think about a success criterion where the students compose the rules of the classroom. This one specific technique allows them to become a part of the school society. It will be a long year and you will need and want buy-in from every student.

Set your goals high and make a student-centered classroom where students take ownership of their learning and mistakes. The best learning will occur from mistakes. Model your mistakes and grow together as a community. A classroom that is safe, fully engaged, and respectful is one where learning is occurring at all times. First and foremost, students want structure. It does not matter where you live in the world. You must be confident and consistent with expectations at all times.

Students need to learn to self-regulate their behaviors. Creating a culture of high performance and respect is not done overnight. One must continue the effort daily with intentional practice. This is where the relationship aspect is crucial. If the students know you believe and care for them, they will do anything. The mentor teacher will come in with support and help in this area of need. One will find he or she is a weathered warrior in this department. Begin to foster this relationship with ongoing support throughout the school year. Get the students to behave, get them to believe.

Management challenges will be ongoing throughout your career. It is important to realize there is not a magic serum. Quite honestly, if the first-year teachers can master one thing it should be management. Without strong management, learning cannot occur successfully.

Many people say we need to crack down on discipline in schools. No matter how much discipline you administer without a relationship, behavior will not change. The most effective management is to get students to cooperate and respect themselves and each other. To commit to cooperate, we must own our behavior. Students must stop blaming and start embracing mistakes. We must be a community where every voice is heard and respected at all times, no matter the circumstances.

Reflections:

- How will you encourage students to be part of the rule process?
- What do high expectations look like to you?
- What will the plan be for fostering a relationship with the mentor?
- Do you truly understand the background and culture of every student?
- Are the students afraid of something or someone?

WHAT ARE WAYS WE CAN TEACH OUR STUDENTS HOW TO BE IN HEALTHY RELATIONSHIPS?

- Encourage students
- Get them involved
- Offer fun and meaningful incentives
- Get creative
- Draw connections from real life
- Become the entertainer of the classroom
- Spark interest and joy
- Laugh more
- Be kinder
- Teach communication skills as a morning routine

Chapter 16

STORY TIME

In a new teacher's classroom many years ago, a young boy moved into the classroom community in early March. The rules and expectations had already been established. The classroom was student-led, and the educator was the effective facilitator. Suddenly, upon the arrival of the new young man, the classroom became chaotic. He was like a tornado throughout the classroom. The educator was unaware of how one student could have such a substantial impact on the classroom. She soon realized the young man was trying his very best to be the comedian in the class.

The teacher pulled him aside and asked if he was an actual comedian who traveled and performed. Well, he looked back at the educator like she was crazy. He quite quickly replied no! The educator asked if he knew Jamie Foxx, the comedian. He replied yes, and the educator told him he had lived in the school district years prior.

The new plan was to help the class lighten up a little bit at the end of the day. He gained permission to spend the last five minutes daily making the class laugh during the lineup. She provided the choice to start that day or wait a few days to get the material ready. The young boy responded that he would practice and be ready.

The educator placed an important rule prior to the agreement. He had to be serious with instruction and wait until the end of class. After that, he was good as gold and could not wait to have his spotlight performance at the end of class to make everyone laugh.

Chapter 17

Scenarios

Throughout the career of an educator, practicing situations will make one better. The absolute truth is, the more a teacher practices, the better they become. The examples below will provide scenarios seen in the classroom. One suggestion would be to make these scenarios part of the new teacher's professional development. Grouping teachers together and providing scenarios for practice will provide intentional time to create strategies and preparedness for the first days.

SCENARIO 1: THE DAILY MEET AND GREET

The daily greeting of students individually at the door will promote success. The first impression is an essential part of the day. A new teacher must understand that students are arriving from locations where they may not matter to anyone. One must make the student realize they count every second of the day. It is imperative to work to get excited when greeting someone. Plan and create a unique manner in which to welcome those one meets. Some examples might be a high five, hug, or knuckle bump. Kids love silly things that get them excited about the day. Many off-task behaviors can be prevented early at the initial greeting of the day.

Now it is time to set up practice. The new educator will practice greeting students individually at the door. Instruct and practice the model to represent different personalities (happy, exuberant, shy, angry/complex). Teachers will design a specific plan for how the students enter the classroom. Create a way to make a positive connection daily, realizing as an adult that we like it when people get excited to see us. When every student has entered the room with a unique greeting, it will be a great day.

SCENARIO 2: GOODBYE RITUAL

The daily goodbye ritual will be necessary at the end of each day. Quite frankly, it may be the last positive thing they hear or see in the day. The new teacher will plan, discuss, and demonstrate a regular daily goodbye ritual. Think about what the verbal signals might consist of positively. Practice with mentor teachers or at the in-service time what this will look like in the classroom. The last seen or heard is carried home and remembered the most.

Think about ways to show one truly cares about each individual in a safe, orderly manner. New teachers will want to leave students wanting more and ready to come back tomorrow. Always remember that everyone deserves a fresh start every day. Sometimes the teacher is all these kids will hold onto in their thoughts.

Scenario 3: Problematic Child/Quiet Child/Discouraged Child

These situations can be frustrating and need reflection from the new teacher. Remember to travel back to the connections made with each student. What does the relationship look like, and how can it become deeper? Are they comfortable talking to the students? How can one motivate them for success? The quicker one takes them to a win, the better. Do they feel essential or invisible? One way to always help someone go to better behavior is to make them laugh—try humor. Now it will be the new teacher's turn to practice engaging with each type of student. Consider some positive language to utilize that may turn the day around. Then, think about ways and actions to deescalate the situation.

Scenario 4: Transitions

The aspect of teaching must have a unique, laid-out plan. The planning component seems to be an area of weakness for many. One must practice traveling from place to place in the quickest manner possible. If a class remains in the hallway too long, the wheels will fall off. New teachers always need a plan. Make clear directions for the actual transition time.

First, one must praise the students who are ready and return to the practice stage for those not quite there. Next, be cautious. It may be a time when a teacher and student voices can become raised. The frustration level can become heightened due to the child pushing buttons and not listening. Finally, one must remain calm and practice. If things are getting out of control, return to the classroom and regroup.

Practice until the students know how to transition safely and productively; only with practice can students become successful. Plan classroom signals and callbacks for this time of transition; at all times make certain that students know what to look for when providing these cues.

Create a classroom success criterion (student contract) with students to build on a positive system in the room. This class contract can occur during the first few days of school. Often one does not think and plan through procedures, and one may react impulsively. Note always to have a plan, do not tell, scaffold and model the process.

The new teacher will now practice this process. Think about what it will look like and how to practice. Check to see if students' understanding is evident and safe at all times. If the plan is not working, reevaluate and try again. Remember to gain the assistance of the mentor and discuss options. Notice that adults have plans for everything, including what they will cook for dinner. Create a good strategy for transitions.

SCENARIO 5: BLURTING OUT IN CLASS

The role-playing activity of a pronounced blurter is one of the most important for a new teacher. The situation can become problematic very quickly. When a few students constantly blurt, it can quickly ruin a lesson. If children are blurting, they may want to have a voice in the discussion. So first, consider the question, why? Once the understanding of the reason makes a deliberate point, pull them aside and discuss any issues they may be having. Work to be on the same page with ideas on how to stop the issue. For example, the speaking chips would be a good resource daily, giving them three chips, and once used up, they cannot speak for the remainder of the time.

The new teacher may assign class roles to create a clear understanding of expectations. Adults want to have a voice and love to communicate. Give opportunities for discussion just as one would like in a meeting or training. Now it is time for the new educator to practice the plan for a blurter. Create and model how one might respond to the situation.

SCENARIO 6: NOT TURNING IN HOMEWORK

It will be imperative to understand the reason behind the action of not turning in homework. The new teacher will not want to revert to the old school ways. Homework should be meaningful if it is going to be assigned. One will not want to create busy work. Life is busy enough for kids and families. If it is quality work and the student is not turning it in, consider some essential questions.

Is it because when he or she goes home, life is out of control? Is it due to laziness? Think about the reasons behind the action. The new teacher will need to remember: that every child is not alike. If the home life is depraved, think of another way to provide practice—possibly first thing in the morning. One might consider the reason behind laziness. Quite possibly, the student is bored, or the assignment is not meaningful. Now is the time for the new teacher to plan, discuss, and model homework. Reflect on class experiences. Did homework help support the student to gain knowledge? Is it just used to create busy work?

SCENARIO 7: MESSY CLASSROOM

New teachers set great intentions early on in the year to keep a tidy classroom. Unfortunately, sometimes these intentions do not come into our practice. Think about the organization and set a weekly time to get items back in order. You will want to be cautious of stacks that become overwhelming.

Possibly, assign jobs so students can assist with keeping items in different set locations. If your room is cluttered and messy, this is most likely a sign that you are out of balance. Work to gain back control. Could you clean it up? Create a game with students, set a timer, and clean rapidly. Remind yourself to check weekly and reflect if you are a tidy role model for students or if an adjustment is necessary. Take the time to plan, discuss, and model ways to keep a clean classroom. Remember to gain support from the administrator or mentor.

SCENARIO 8: FAILING STUDENTS

New teachers never set out to encounter failure. However, sometimes students come to the classroom behind and cannot do the work efficiently and correctly. Often the students do not understand the content. A plan must be set into place to handle these types of situations. One must first check the district policy for grading.

Be alert to notifying the parents early on in the year. Notice that if a student is failing, there is a reason behind it. Do not wait to enter the grades in the grade book until the last minute. A teacher may find they do not have enough grades for an individual and become panicked. Quite often, a district may have a minimum requirement for each subject.

Remember, the new teacher's responsibility must make it a mission to discover the reason behind the failure. Now take the time to reflect on the questions and create a plan, discuss, and model.

- What will the response look like for a failing student?
- Does the student understand the goal?
- What kind of relationship does the teacher have with this student?
- What motivates this kind of student?
- How can one support academics?
- What kind of remedial tutoring or small group could the teacher plan for support?
- Does the teacher need to gain support from a mentor or administrator?

SCENARIO 9: ABSENTEEISM

Students consistently being absent from school will create an alarm for any new educator. However, one must realize it is not always up to the student how they get to school. As adults, one can understand things happen, and educators must find ways to check in more often. Do not wait until numerous days add up; meet with the administrators and notify the parents to find out the problem. Reach out and make contact on the second day the student is absent. Do not rely solely on emails, as sometimes these are not valid. Instead, make the connection through a phone call. Work with the front office to make certain the number is correct for the student.

Take a few moments to reflect on these questions:

- Is this truly the child's fault or is it a situation that may be occurring?
- What is going on at home that is preventing the student from not attending?
- How can one support the change of behavior?

Now, the new teachers turn to plan, discuss, and model a situation of a student being absent and the response.

SCENARIO 10: TALKING BACK/SASSY

As a new teacher, one is sometimes not prepared for the harsh words a child may speak. It is a time when frustration levels can reach an all-time high. Words can hurt, and one can feel out of control. Remember, a child wants to be heard in all aspects of life. Some are coming from places where a role model is not evident. Take the time to have a one-on-one and work to get to the root of the problem. It may be a case in which the student is trying to gain attention. Sometimes extra time will fix this problem. Remember, do not take things so personally; possibly, students may not feel seen or heard. Instead, plan, discuss, and model what it looks like to remain respectful in the classroom.

What will it look like to be the educator who shows and represents the correct way to speak with others?

SCENARIO 11: DISRESPECT

One may find students lack respect in the classroom. It will be essential to teach students how to communicate respectfully in class. New teachers will need to form a community or family within the class. A significant understanding is that a lack of respect will not be accepted. Initially, modeling what it looks like for the teacher and classmates will be imperative. It will be essential to stay positive and calm in all situations of disrespect.

There may be days in which this triggers and stresses one out. Remember to breathe and practice the strategies to be successful. One way that may be helpful is to read stories about respect. A positive classroom may be uncomfortable for some students that thrive in a distressed world.

Continue to utilize the words of safety to students. New teachers will now plan, discuss, and model a student being disrespectful and how one will respond. Correct responses may need to be well-planned thoroughly. Often practicing questions with a mentor or the team can be beneficial.

- How are things at home with the student?
- Have there been any changes?
- What is one noticing?
- What does peer interaction look like at school?
- How is the bus for the child?
- How can one support them in more success?

SCENARIO 12: STUDENT FALLING ASLEEP

Many new educators may find this to push buttons when they are trying to present a powerful lesson. They must remember this is about the child, not themselves. Strategies to implement will be to reach out to the counselor and ask probing questions. Contact the parent or caregiver immediately. Honestly, a parent might not even realize the child is not going to bed on time. Communicate with all parties the concern. Do not shame the child; allow a bit of rest if necessary. Remind yourself that off days are necessary when one does not get rest, even as an adult. New educators plan, discuss, and model the type of student who falls asleep.

SCENARIO 13: FIGHTING

The new teacher will never have the tools for a fight. Therefore, the number one strategy is to react quickly. First, remove other students from the situation. Then, call for help or support, and try and deescalate the situation the best one can. In this situation, one must send the students to the office due to safety issues.

Some widespread first-year responses to issues might become the best choice. It may be pulling the trigger and adding more of a problem to the situation. Some examples follow:

- Call the parents: remember, a teacher must build a relationship in order to relay the difficult information.
- Send to the principal's office: *remember* that the teacher loses all authority at this point. Only send for safety support.
- Assign a student a zero: understand a student will have nowhere to go from this point; defeat will never regain momentum.
- Make him sit by himself during class. This only isolates the student and sometimes promotes more misbehavior.
- Student sitting outside a classroom for a consequence. This may cause alienation for the student and create an unsafe space where a child is not monitored.
- Ten-minute loss of recess for not doing the work. Earlier it was discussed that research does not support the removal of movement as a consequence for misbehavior.
- Give him or her some kind of reward or incentive for making better choices. It is best for the student to learn to motivate themselves and feel good about the correct choices.

Tips:

- Dig deeper into the real problem. The first step is trying to figure out what is going on in the student's life.
- Possibly a student could be having a social issue.

- Is it possible the work is too hard or too easy?
- Is it possible something happened at home in the morning?
- Is it possible it is a friend issue?

Try to get to the bottom of the issue before reacting. It is always better to handle it in the classroom—partner with parents early in the year. Even low socioeconomic parents and grandparents will get involved.

Students like to learn about the world they live in through exciting experiences. Unfortunately, sometimes teachers fall into the act of telling them what to do. Once the new teacher falls into negative behavior, it will take the learning out of the equation. As we have discussed previously, it is crucial not to be reactive in any situation, especially in classroom management.

New teachers must anticipate what might occur before entering the classroom on the first day. Thinking and reflecting on what might be the underlying cause of the situation will promote success. Always remember that one's team can support in these areas. Do not be afraid to ask for help. There are many resources available to provide support. Remember, though, once the management is gone in a classroom, it is challenging to gain it back.

If one stays in the positive circle, one will reach each child with success. It is not about *control;* it is always about the relationship and respect. It is crucial to understand that encouragement and reinforcement of good behavior are essential. It is vital to be descriptive and specific with children. Recognizing work ethic and respect and areas of improvement are always praiseworthy.

SCENARIO 14: REFERRAL PROCESS

What will the steps for the referral process look like? How will one study before school starts? Practice with the specific administrators and look at the specific steps that one will need to follow. Understand that it is important not to self-diagnose a student with learning difficulties. There are steps to follow and additional support to consult along the way.

SCENARIO 15: RUNNER OR STUDENT TRYING TO ESCAPE THE CLASSROOM

Understand the process if a student begins to feel contained and suddenly runs out of the classroom, such as notifying the principal or assistant principal immediately. Try finding a safe place in the classroom for a student to cool off or have the time to return to being a successful student.

SCENARIO 16: DEALING WITH AN INATTENTIVE STUDENT

Many students may not be disruptive, but they seem nonattentive and checked out of the lesson. Teachers may want to try and make eye contact and then possibly pull them back with a question or check to see if they need a moment to be more active.

Remember, as you travel through these different scenarios, do not take the situations to a personal level. Remain calm at all times; do not seem impatient, upset, or irritated with a loud voice or wild body gestures. If the educator remains composed, the situation will deescalate sooner. Often, a teacher can explain a decision to a student, and if they can truly understand the reason, they will get back on track. Never use threats on children, never kick a child out of the classroom, and the teacher should never leave children unattended. Keep a trail of documentation available to back up the decisions in the room.

SCENARIO 17: SCHOOL OR SUPPLY MISUSE

Understand what the protocols are for misuse of property. Discuss damages with the parents and partner up with them to gain a partnership for respect.

SCENARIO 18: CHILDREN BRUISED OR SEEMINGLY IN DISTRESS

Gain contact with the counselor and understand the obligations and protocol for reporting abuse issues. Remember to always have the child's best interest at the forefront of every decision.

Throughout the scenarios, one has learned to practice and become more knowledgeable to perform better in the first year. The new teacher will remove all fear, take the positive initiative, and reflect on how the practice has prepared them for each situation.

Reflections:

- Is there an understanding of all district protocols in the situations?
- How might your actions as a new teacher be perceived by your class, co-workers, and administration?

- How can you impact learning from a certain action for your students in a respectful manner?
- What will you learn to praise, and more often, in a specific manner?

STORY TIME

A student in a class was not turning in his homework. The teacher pulled him to the back table one afternoon early in August while others were at recess. He began to tell the teacher his mother would throw it away every night. She wanted him to do chores, not his schoolwork. The educator came up with an early morning contract to do his homework first thing in the morning. The point of this story is that one never knows what a child might be experiencing or expected to do outside the classroom. Please do not assume it is intentional behavior.

Chapter 18

Feedback

Feedback is a game changer in education. The purpose of feedback is to aid in the learning process and improve academic achievement. In addition, it should provide students with the ability to believe they can achieve success. Therefore, novice educators must gain accurate, effective, and efficient feedback to evaluate ongoing understanding.

Feedback will progress from the surface level to assist students for their learning. Gaining an understanding that prompts can support effective feedback will be necessary. Feedforward differs from feedback. It replaces positive or negative feedback with looking more toward future solutions. In this type of feedback, suggestions, recommendations, and encouragement will occur. The support provides a person with a chance to own their behavior and work toward excellence.

John Hattie defines feedback as the "information provided by an agent (e.g., teacher, peer, book, parent, self, experience) regarding aspects of one's performance understanding," and is the consequence of a person's performance. Examples from Hattie's work will support the new teacher with knowing how to give the specific feedback or feedforward needed for ongoing success.[1]

When a student begins to look at the feedforward method and take ownership, the shift in learning occurs to actual ownership: the student's understanding of where they are going and how they are going to get there. Frequently, a rubric can be beneficial for the students.

When the student takes ownership in the learning process, it will provide achievement and an ongoing yearly transfer. Furthermore as, the learner has clear expectations of the learning, greater automaticity will occur to complete the task.

Additionally, according to Hattie, feedback may differ according to its level of cognitive complexity: It can refer to a task, a process, or one's self-regulation. Task-level feedback means that someone receives feedback about the content, facts, or surface information. For example, how well have the tasks been completed and understood? Is the result of a task correct or incorrect? Feedback at the process level means that a person receives feedback on the strategies of his or her performance. Feedback at this level aims to process information that is necessary to understand or complete a specific task. What needs to be understood and mastered with the tasks?

Feedback at the level of self-regulation means that someone receives feedback about the individual's regulation of the strategies they are using for their performance. In contrast to process level feedback, feedback on this level does not provide information on choosing or developing strategies but monitors the use of strategies of the learning process. It aims at a more remarkable skill in self-evaluation or confidence to engage further on a task (What can be done to manage, guide, and monitor your way of action?).

The self-level focuses on the personal characteristics of the feedback recipient (often praise about the person). One of the arguments about the variability is that feedback needs to focus on the appropriate question and level of cognitive complexity. If not, the message can easily be ignored, misunderstood, and be of low value to the recipient.

Students and adults thrive with specific feedback. One must be intentional and understand the appropriate ways in which to give feedback. One concern in the area of feedback is that one is cautious not to make a competitive instrument. It should be an individual response for each child. Be mindful about the students' own personal best; everyone is unique and has different talents. Another area of caution is for the student not to feel like the feedback is controlling them. Students love to have ownership in every task and attempt.

Lastly, do not overdo feedback with all positive. The new educator will need to be genuine and remember specifics with feedback. For example, when giving feedback, is it genuinely triggering the students to think harder? Is the learning going deeper?

Note that this process will take practice and time to understand this technique. So be mindful and put in the time; the benefits will be rewarding, and the students will own their part in the process. Notice along the way feedback provides value. Value creates self-worth; self-worth builds futures.

Table 18.1 shows examples of John Hattie's research.

Management can also be supported by redirecting inappropriate behavior with correct real-time feedback. New educators must remain calm and take the student aside to feel safe. Express the feeling calmly and identify inappropriate behavior. Sometimes a student just needs a few moments to gain the control back. Let the student sit and have a moment of peace. It is the adult who needs to always have composure over the situation. Stay in your positive circle reflecting on what feedback is appropriate for every situation. Finding a mentor with which to practice the feedback situations will be helpful.

Table 18.1 Examples of John Hattie's Research.

Task level	Task level is focused on how well the task is being accomplished or performed. Feedback might include distinguishing correct from incorrect information, and/or building more surface knowledge.	Does the student's answer meet the success criteria? Is the student correct/incorrect? How well can the student elaborate on the answer? What is the correct answer? What other information is needed to meet the criteria?
Process level	This level of feedback is specific to the process underlying the tasks or relating and extending tasks. Such feedback includes relationships among ideas, strategies or error detection, explicitly learning from errors, and/or cuing the learner to different strategies and errors.	What strategies did the student use? What other questions can the student ask about the task? What are the relationships with other parts of the task? What is the student's understanding of concept/ knowledge related to the task?
Self-Regulation	This type of feedback supports students to monitor, direct, and regulate action towards the learning goal. Feedback might include the ability to create internal feedback and to self-assess and/or seeking to help find further information and/or confirm a response.	How can the student monitor the work? How can the student carry out self-checking? What does the information have in common? How have their ideas changed? Can the student teach another student how to?

Source: Hattie and Timperley, 2007.

Behavior needs feedback and plans for solutions often. Quite frankly, sometimes the teachers need the moments as well. Go ahead and take that deep breath. Most likely, the child and maybe even the teacher will be embarrassed by the situation. Let them sit and have a moment of peace. There may be occasions when a student may have an outburst and not understand their behavior. At this time, it will be important to point out the problem with correct, thought-out feedback and travel to a solution with respect and possibilities. Listen and travel to the positive circle together; a solution will occur.

Proper respect with the correct feedback does not just happen automatically for a new educator. It will take time and practice with this framework of thinking. Refrain from the negative criticism. Truly no human enjoys these kinds of remarks. Most of the time, everyone will shut down with negative feedback and not continue to grow. Frequently it creates and promotes learned helplessness, and one shuts down and gives up. Some tools to provide feedback may be to utilize Post-it Notes for quick private feedback, invite the student to give other students quality feedback, or hold a one-on-one conference with the student to hear comments and set goals for moving forward.

Remember, students can make significant gains when ownership is valued, and everyone knows when they are meeting expectations. Students benefit from hearing the feedback and coming up with a plan of action and how the behaviors are increasing learning. It will be necessary not to give vague comments and responses because these become ineffective. Instead, it is vital to be specific with the problem and support a plan of action. Seek out the solution at all times.

Reflections:

- Could you possibly lead the class on this specific teaching point?
- By understanding the problem, you are closer to meeting your goal.
- Everyone is using intelligent voices and making the correct decision.
- You see the problem now; how can you change the behavior for a better solution?
- How has your thought changed from the beginning until now?

STORY TIME

A teacher is reminded of her childhood when she gave a speech in a class. She had worked long hours on the assignment to provide quality work. The speech was given, and her teacher gave all negative comments in front of her peers. This experience impacted her public speaking throughout her education. She worked diligently through the years to move past her public speaking fears. From this experience, she realized how powerful feedback could be. The lesson takeaway was never to allow her students to feel this way.

NOTE

1. Hattie, John, and Helen Timperley. "The Power of Feedback." *Review of Educational Research* 77, no. 1 (March 2007): 81–112. https://doi.org/10.3102/003465430298487.

Chapter 19

Parent Communication

In college, one has studied theory and listened to lectures about parental support. Once the teaching practice, observation, and modeling occur in a safe atmosphere, the transfer can occur. The goal is to carry this practice in an effective manner into the classroom.

Let's begin to think wiser and smarter about our practice. Embrace flexibility to adjust to difficult situations in our first year. Overcome our doubts and fears, letting go of those items that are not serving us well in our daily lives. Why is it important to communicate with parents successfully? Parents are the first educators in a child's eyes. Teachers must respect and understand that the belief system has been established. Teachers must earn the respect and support of parents. You must not assume they will respect you just because you are a teacher.

General ideas for meeting parents:

- Listen more and talk less—listen to hear, don't listen to respond.
- Be positive and hopeful.
- Act confident yet humble, not a know-it-all.
- Avoid education jargon and acronyms.

Never promise anything you or the school cannot deliver. It is always okay to say one needs to check on something before offering a definite answer. Utilize the phrase "Good question, I will get back to soon with the answer." Utilize the phrase, "I understand" because you are a good listener with parents. Be conscious and avoid the word *but;* it can foster confrontation. New teachers must learn to sit quietly and not interrupt. In the reality of the situation, parents can be such a great asset to a child's education.

Effective teachers pursue partnerships with parents and families in a professional manner for the benefit of students. It may be very difficult for new teachers if they are younger and do not have children of their own.

Many new teachers are not equipped right out of college to deal with some of the understandings of all children or parental situations. It will be necessary to recognize the parents are very protective of their sweet babies. In most eyes, they can do no wrong, so when they do, it can take on a true battle-like form. Parents often come from a place where a school was not a positive place.

As educators, we must be prepared to not escalate a situation with the manner in which we approach it. One way to support a new teacher is to role-play these scenarios. In some cases, this will actually alleviate a lot of stress that will occur at the beginning of the year.

WHAT IS EFFECTIVE PARENT COMMUNICATION?

Think about the following:

- What are the needs, and how can you support this individual parent the most? Do they need additional resources?
- What is the purpose of the discussion? Remember: both parties have a love for the child and want what is best. Make sure the parent truly understands the purpose of the discussion.
- How does the schedule work for everyone involved? This can be difficult. We must support and try and communicate when best for a parent. Do not give up if you cannot initially schedule a meeting. Keep trying and be persistent.
- How are both parties being active listeners? Remember to hear what the parent has to say—really try to understand. Putting yourself in their shoes sometimes will help, especially if you do not have children of your own.
- How is the new educator keeping a positive tone? Always, always have a positive tone—even if a parent voice escalates.
- It is okay to tell a parent that you need to reschedule with an administrator present.
- New teachers should never feel threatened or in an unsafe situation.

WHY IS PARENT COMMUNICATION BENEFICIAL?

- Drives strong relationships in your classroom
- Increases trust among all
- Encourages higher and realistic parental expectations
- Increases home/school connection—shows you care

Early on, build the relationship by encouraging a commitment between parent, student, and teacher. It will be crucial to be aware of different communication approaches. As educators, one must recognize how different approaches can strengthen or weaken parent/teacher relationships. New teachers must gain practice in employing different communication approaches in all circumstances. It is important to create an awareness of topics that should be communicated. Some examples are academic performance, behavioral performance, social skills, and health-related issues.

As new professionals travel through the year, many may experience barriers in communication. Some examples are the public perspective shared on media sites or cultural differences. It will be important to understand the culture of the child and respect their beliefs.

Parents' perspectives of the school may be tarnished because of the way they grew up. Economics and school language can play a role in which a parent relates to a teacher. It is important to formulate a plan on how you will take action when each of these challenges begins to occur. Practicing and reflecting will allow one's formulated plan to go successfully with parent conferences.

Many times, parents will need guidance and support. Sometimes this is difficult for a new teacher who might not have children of their own. Listed below are ways in which we can educate on responsibility and respect. The number one item to remember is to remind parents to be involved in their child's education and accept parental responsibilities with open communication.

One needs to be aware of protocols. For example, know your building rules on window covers; parents might want to watch the class. Know the expectations of parents in the hallway before, during, and after school. Have parents email to set up a conference and reply with wanting to know their concerns to address; this will allow preparation.

Often new teachers wonder how parents may react to their child's account of a situation. Parents will and always will take the child's side in the situation. Be cautious about how to approach correctly to keep a solid team with parents. You must allow parents to see the professional and personal side of you as well. They are trying to make a connection. Sometimes it might seem as if you are helping to support and raise them as well. It will be necessary to form a plan to get to know them prior to an incident with their child. I recommend calling and bragging about outstanding things prior to the negative.

Parents love success in their children. Phone calls to parents can be very intimidating, so our first role play will focus on the first phone call home. Hopefully, you have already established contact at a meet the new teacher night in which you have at least been able to spend a few moments with them to build a start of a relationship.

What Is Your Plan of Action for Initial Parent Contact?

- Transportation (very important prior to school and make it aware of necessary changes)
- Plan the back-to-school night
- Plan grade-level parent meetings; this can be a team effort—safety in numbers
- Plan letters home; do not bombard with too much information
- Plan phone calls during the first week
- Plan notes home during the first week

Some fun ideas might be to make copies of some of the positive letters and mail them to the child when they graduate from high school. Reminder: never mail the negative responses; you may get one of these every so often.

What Is Your Plan for Communication with Parents Throughout the Year?

- Plan a classroom newsletter
- Plan invitations to group presentations
- Plan one positive note home every day
- Plan student-made invitations to schoolwide functions

Begin the year by pairing up new teachers and create a list of what one wishes parents would do this year and what one wishes to do as an educator. This activity will allow new teachers to reflect on the importance of this critical relationship. Work to make connections early in the year with parents. It will be the best bonding technique in the new relationship.

There will never be a moment when over-communication happens with parents. The more they are informed the better the partnerships will become. Parents are starting the school year in the positive circle. It is a fresh start for the parents just like the child. Remind all parties it is a year to enjoy success.

- How will you keep building the relationship in a positive manner?
- What does your plan look like?

BUILDING THE INITIAL RELATIONSHIP

Role Play/Practice

Remember, practice is one of the best ways a new teacher can prepare for the new year. It is crucial to focus on the first phone call as getting to know the parent and opening the lines of communication. You will want to convey enthusiasm about the child and refrain from all negative comments. The new teacher can be supported by practicing the first phone call with an administrator, mentor, or another new teacher.

The first phone call should happen soon in the year. Remember to take time to know something about the student prior to the phone call. This will allow the new teacher to establish a positive team relationship with the parent that can flourish throughout the school year. It is important to understand that the parent must know that you have the child's best interest at heart with every aspect from being safe, emotional, and educational. Work to truly see that one is genuine and honest in the relationship.

Reflections:

- How will you stay on the topic of conversation?
- What message do you want to convey?
- What do you want to have to happen as a result of this communication?
- Plan a manner in which you will communicate early about problems.
- Plan the act of performing as a professional at all times.
- Plan to understand and respect the rights and efforts of parents/guardians.

STORY TIME

A new teacher reflected on the compliment given by a parent. The parent was so grateful that the teacher knew how precious their time was with a busy schedule. She was specific about her concerns and gave concrete examples of her student's work. The parent stated the new teacher always listened, and they brainstormed solutions together. It was a significant relationship in which they felt as though it was a partnership from the beginning.

Chapter 20

Parent–Teacher Conference

Teachers will need to outline the topics that will be necessary to discuss and make a detailed plan. Check with the administrator on how to make sure the topics are correct. It will be important to have notes on student work, assessment results, child development, and anything else necessary to share. Remember to begin with the positive, good things.

Having the parents sit across from you is not a wise idea. Sitting across from one another can foster or breed adversarial confrontation that most often backfires. Sometimes the situations are severely not resolved. Let's be honest, no parent wants to sit at a small child's desk and speak to another adult. Be respectful of parents' time, comfort, and topics.

Stay on track with the meeting. Keep a timer so that you remain on track. Five-minute opening: say something positive (yes, there is something positive about each child—find it!). Ten-minute report on academics: stay on topic—it is about the evidence. Five-minute summary: wrap up with the positive—remember, it is a partnership—and thank them for the time investment.

If notes are necessary, take them to support the future growth of the student. Read the body language of the parent. If it is escalating excuse yourself and get support. Mind your body language. Do not sit with your arms crossed. Again, sit them next to you or at a round table.

If more time is needed, schedule a follow-up to go into more detail about the topics needed. Prepare a few introductory questions to begin speaking with the parents. Prepare to be a good listener from the start. Remind parents you are a partnership. Remember to always go to the positive circle. Try not to just focus on a list of negative items. Remember, you are allowed reflection time and so are the parents.

The new teacher must be prepared for any surprises that may arise. Sometimes parents will travel to the negative realm very quickly. One may hear them describing their own child in a negative light. It will be important to intervene with positives and support them in traveling back to the positive quickly. If the parents are struggling with personal problems, support when you can but remember that your main focus is the child. Avoid the word *but* and stick to the facts—no negative emotions, no promises. Stay in your positive circle using kind words about the child. Remember, both parties should be centered around love and safety for children.

The profession is one that the new teacher enters like a chosen extraordinary gift. When one can focus on different perspectives and center on possibilities for a child's future, success will occur. One can enhance the ability to stay positive for longer periods of time. Our actions of the day are often a result of our approach and belief systems. Reflect on the process of not being afraid to be open with a parent. If the relationship is built, one can be personable and realistic. Keep in mind ways to make a difference and support parents in developing and growing their children.

As you travel throughout the school year you may see some different styles of parenting and be in need of tips and tricks. The helicopter parent is one that is always peering through the window of the classroom. This kind of parent may challenge the grading at times and does not like the child to suffer or struggle with any situations. Parents might not want consequences or actions taken with their children. These parents sometimes believe their child deserves special treatment or privileges. It will be the new teacher's responsibility to understand the grading policies for the district. Be sure you are aligned with the team and do not be a grading outlier.

Some parents will truly believe their child is first in everything and oftentimes have unrealistic views of the child. Some helpful ideas will be to listen and be clear about standards for all children. Often reference school policy when speaking about concerns. Send home enrichment work and allow the parent to be involved at the correct times. Allow areas in which the parents can assist and feel needed. Oftentimes these parents are first-time school parents.

Be cautious of parents who want to hold conferences in the pickup lane, hallway, grocery store, and athletic games. One tip is to quietly ask the parent to email you with concerns and tell them you will get back to them promptly to schedule a conference. Understand school building expectations for parents in the building. Oftentimes new teachers become frustrated from lack of communication. These might not show up for conferences or answer any phone calls.

Understanding early about the different types of parents is helpful. Know your audience. Single parents or grandparents need extra support. Understanding the situation might be very difficult. Some could be unemployed or work odd hours. Are they battling a medical condition? Are they incarcerated? The list goes on and on. The bottom line is to know your audience. Some suggestions are to try and have empathy. Modify the schedule if necessary and accommodate when at all possible. Document these situations so one has a good record of attempts to contact. Do not give up trying and never punish a child for lack of involvement.

Another caution in supporting parents is to maintain boundaries and professionalism. Some parents might feel comfortable calling you at home, wanting personal information. They visit daily, bring treats, and want to discuss all the children in the classroom. You must remember to enforce boundaries between what is appropriate and inappropriate. Have them call you Mr. or Ms. at all times, stay on topic during conferences, and always keep the focus on the student.

Some parents may be the type that will blame or name call. They will not accept any accountability and all problems are a result of you the new teacher. Some comments may be that the child never had any problems prior to this class, or they want you to be the fixer of all social and academic problems. Some suggestions will be to keep plenty of documentation. Work with the mentor to give you feedback. Never meet with these parents alone; utilize your team or an administrator for extra support.

Sometimes as a new teacher it is difficult to come up with affirmations for the special student. New teachers must make an intentional habit of giving positive affirmations. Students will thrive when they feel good about themselves just as a new teacher will thrive. In education, teachers are underappreciated. Coaches, administrators, and mentors will work to give positive accolades to new educators. It will be necessary to make it a point to give students and quite possibly parents positive feedback.

Positivity draws you to the next level of success. Pause a moment, look around, and see the positive side of everything. Your positive circle is full of love, commitment, grit, and possibilities. Do not let the positivity fade. Remember, many days this takes work; put in the hard work. The return on investment will be sizeable. Listed below are some ideas that will guide you throughout the year. They will strengthen self-esteem and last a lifetime.

One must build trust with the parent. Continue to describe that we value respect in our classroom and that partnership is important. Work to fix the issues. One recommendation is to sit down as a team, the child and parent, so that everyone knows you are working for the greater good. Remember to view the parent as a partner, remembering they loved them first.

AFFIRMATION EXAMPLES

- ____ is eager and participates energetically in class.
- ____ is diligent and focused at everything they attempt.
- ____ is a cheerful student but still struggles on ___ attempting to move to solution.

- _____ has a great energy about school.
- _____ shows attentiveness in ____subject and is showing success.

It will be imperative to share with parents to provide the help and encouragement at home to support their child.

Reflections:

- What will your choice of two affirmations to utilize this week look like?
- Do you need to repair a relationship or admit a mistake?
- How has building a relationship with every parent shifted your practice to positive?

STORY TIME

A new teacher began to reflect on a parent who burst into tears during a meeting. The parent explained that she was going through a tough divorce and how much her child loved school. She stated it was the only thing she did not have to worry about in this entire process. She knew her son was in good hands during the day.

Chapter 21

Midyear Rejuvenation

As the weather gets cooler and the holidays approach excitement may fill the air. School buildings are decorated, laughter is heard in the hallway, and students are celebrating with gift exchanges and parties. But quite honestly, stress can be higher than ever before. Students may not feel the same excitement in the air. Some children may be on edge due to returning to an environment where basic needs are neglected and not met. Students may begin to show discipline problems. The students realize that one stable person will not be around for two weeks or more. So they will need a lot of reassurance at this point before the break.

Once all the students head home, the new teacher can take a deep breath. Traveling into the holiday, reflect and organize prior to leaving. Listen to what the body truly needs. Reality sets in that those two weeks away from the building have finally arrived.

Hopes spill into hearts that quite possibly, a new teacher might be made to fulfill this special destiny. This time of year, you have been striving to be a master at working, planning, designing, creating, and performing daily at high levels. Recharge, gain rest, and enable your thoughts to climb the mountain. Return with a plan to be ready to conquer the remainder of the year.

When you return in January, remember not to pretend you have everything under control. Reach out and find the support needed to finish the year. You must verbalize when you are struggling. Reminding again, you are not at a loss; is it normal to need extra support. You should not want to settle for less. Stay pumped up and ready to conquer in the first year.

Reflections:

- Have you written down the answers to the midyear checklist?
- Is there an area that needs more work?
- What can be celebrated at this moment?

Table 21.1 Midyear Checklist

What are some personal strengths at this mid-point in the year? How can one celebrate them and make a note of them?	Ways That Show	What Is Next?
What does one's classroom culture look like? How can one improve relationships in all areas? Does one need to restructure something? How is one's health? How is one planning for some personal fun? How will one bring joy to the classroom and beyond daily? What is one grateful for at this moment? What is something that is going well in the classroom? What fun activity has one participated in lately just for oneself? What has one achieved lately? How is one respecting oneself and others? What does one need to abandon? What does one need to keep doing? How is one revisiting the systems? How is one keeping organized? What is the plan to purge and clean the different areas? How will one sort piles? Which areas need the most attention? Have has one found one thing to love about each student? Does one really know all the names?		

STORY TIME

This new teacher was stressed out midyear and trying to pull herself together to walk through the classroom. She wiped tears away throughout the school day. She realized she was comparing herself to other perfect teachers. Her environment felt toxic. She decided to tell her principal she would be leaving her position. The new teacher discussed some options and support. She decided to take care of herself over the break. The return was a success, and she finished very strong with no regrets. Her lesson was not to take on so much and utilize the tips for beating stress better in her life. She found the balance needed to continue and was very glad she did not give up easily.

Chapter 22

Student Engagement

According to the *Glossary of Education Reform*, student engagement "refers to the degree of attention, curiosity, interest, optimism, and passion that students show when they are learning or being taught, which extends to the level of motivation they have to learn and progress in their education."[1]

The authentically engaged student usually:

- Loves learning because it is meaningful and makes sense.
- Immerses in the work and finds value.
- Strives to earn an exemplary grade and most likely will make it happen.
- Strives to get into a college and be successful in the world.
- Volunteers and gives feedback to the teachers and peers.
- Remembers the learning from year to year.

It is essential to understand that children gain excitement when they are interested and participating in a lesson. Effective learning occurs, and a sense of belonging when goals are clear, and the students are a big part of this practice from the start. An engaged, active class does not mean an out-of-control class. It is the way students react to the work.

Engagement for the new teacher will make for a more exciting classroom and bring a specific type of joy. It is crucial to be able to recognize student thinking and doing when it is occurring. The new teacher's directions must be clear and in language that is understood. The manner in which a new teacher changes the voice intonation can play a huge role in engagement. Sometimes a mere whisper can gain the attention of a lesson.

At times just kneeling at the level of students and looking them eye to eye will promote the engagement component. Include student names periodically to help hook the learning. Students sometimes need to be encouraged to participate in the lesson. When students feel confident, they will try new skills and be eager to participate. The difference is glaring between strategically compliant and genuinely engaged in the work.

Many strategies can be incorporated in the classroom to engage students in activities. Creating more personalized work allows students to benefit greatly. Pacing will also be important in the lesson structure so that students do not become overwhelmed or bored. A reminder needed often is that the teacher is the facilitator in the classroom. If the new teacher is going home more tired than students, something is wrong.

Make sure at all times materials are well planned and prepared. Teachers do not get in the habit of commenting on every little thing that students are doing with off-task behavior. Often technology can play a role in student engagement. For example, students today enjoy the game-like atmosphere. They may also allow for the hands-on component in the classroom where students can produce while thinking and questioning will increase the level.

The best suggestion for a new teacher is not to try too many new tricks at first. Add to one's toolbox slowly and grasp a few things at a time. Engagement in the classroom is often difficult to monitor. The new educator needs to work on the small-group instruction, briefly introducing and then pulling the small group to engage in the lesson.

The new teacher will often see the veteran teacher always having students' eyes and attention. It could feel disheartening to a new educator. Remind yourself not to feel embarrassed or unnerved. The engagement component will come with time and practice. Begin to reflect on how to gain students' support with daily tasks. We learned earlier one must become actively involved in growing. Learn early to become a self-directed learner, and search out professional development tools for engagement. There are many techniques to try. Then, when you continue to grow and understand the engagement of lessons, stay positive, and learning will become very fulfilling for you and your students.

Reflections:

- Are students truly paying attention to the lesson at hand?
- Are students taking notes and discussing topics?
- Do the students feel a sense of ownership in the lesson?
- Can the students articulate the job at hand with interest?
- Do the students have set goals and are they working to deepen knowledge daily?

STORY TIME

The teacher reflected that the students felt comfortable and were doing even more than she thought possible. Both teacher and students felt a partnership.

She always tried to put herself in the students' shoes when planning the lessons. She felt their appreciation when she planned with them on her shoulders.

NOTE

1. *The Glossary of Education Reform*. Accessed July 5, 2021. https://www.edglossary.org/.

Chapter 23

Gratitude and Educators

In the next chapter, we will understand why we must be grateful that we have persevered this far. We have taken all the tips and practiced and gained support. When one understands gratitude, it can have a dramatic and lasting effect on a person's life, said Robert A. Emmons, professor of psychology at the University of California, Davis, and a leading scientific expert on the science of gratitude.

The nature and importance of gratitude have been studied in psychology today. It has indicated that gratitude can improve well-being in two ways: directly, as a causal agent of well-being, and indirectly, as a means of buffering against negative states and emotions. Gratitude research can amplify thinking within current theoretical models, including both cognitive-behavioral and person-centered approaches. Gratitude can enhance the well-being of a person.

Emmons believes gratitude works because it allows individuals to celebrate the present and be active participants in their own lives. Begin to value and appreciate friends, oneself, situations, and circumstances, and focused on what an individual already has rather than something absent or a need is emphasized in his research. In education and life, one has many things to be grateful for throughout the first year. New teachers must enhance their well-being throughout the mission.

One will need to reflect on how and when to be grateful. Gratitude is essential even when one is overwhelmed. If nothing else, be grateful for a job. Some, unfortunately, are waking up in the world jobless and hungry today. It is a choice; choose wisely.

In the following template, the new teacher can take the time to reflect and center oneself back on positivity. Take a few moments to reflect on the gratitude questionnaire. It will allow teachers to see areas that might need to be redirected toward a healthier, more grateful mindset.

The Gratitude Questionnaire—Six Item Form (GQ-6) By Michael E. McCullough, Ph.D., Robert A. Emmons, Ph.D., Jo-Ann Tsang, Ph.D.

Using the scale below as a guide, write a number beside each statement to indicate how much you agree with it.

1 = strongly disagree	**2** = disagree
3 = slightly disagree	**4** = neutral
5 = slightly agree	**6** = agree
7 = strongly agree	

____1. I have so much in life to be thankful for.

____2. If I had to list everything that I felt grateful for, it would be a very long list.

____3. When I look at the world, I don't see much to be grateful for.*

____4. I am grateful to a wide variety of people.

____5. As I get older I find myself more capable to appreciate the people, events, and situations that have been part of my life history.

____6. Long amounts of time can go by before I feel grateful to something or someone.*

* Items 3 and 6 are reverse-scored

Reflections:

- Did any answers come as a surprise?
- How can you begin to have more gratitude?
- Do you truly understand how important gratitude is in education?

STORY TIME

A new educator realized something was not right with her student. She decided to follow her heart and see what was happening behind the scenes. She soon discovered the student's sole caregiver, her mother, had lost her job. The educator collected canned goods and warm jackets for the family. One afternoon she delivered the merchandise to the family with a smile. She realized there was a lot to be grateful for in her own life.

NOTE

1. McCullough, Michael E., Robert A. Emmons, and Jo-Ann Tsang. "Penn Institute Gratitude Questionnaire—Social Skills Plus." Social Skills Plus. Accessed November 10, 2021. https://socialskillsplus.com/wp-content/uploads/2018/11/Penn-Institute-Gratitude-Questionnaire.pdf.

Chapter 24

End of the Year

The days are getting hotter and longer while the students are getting more chaotic, rambunctious, and just downright squirrely. It is springtime, and everything is blooming. Often the rain is moving in and canceling recess. Teachers and students are sneezing and wheezing. New teachers are highly exhausted and feel like they cannot go on another day. The alarm clock goes off, and you sigh deeply and think to yourself, it is quite possible; "I cannot go on another day in education." Nevertheless, dig deep and set a mindset to finish strong. These students need the teachers to show up every day, even to the end.

When the first year begins to end and testing time is upon the horizon, do not forget how you have arrived at this place. Look over at the boy who is sitting worried at his desk and be there for him. You will begin to look back at this year and ask, did you merely endure or truly touch lives? The end of the year is valuable time, so do not waste it. Students and teammates may drive you crazy in the end days. Some children are headed home to chaos, and the school remains the only safe place for them. Unfortunately, children will travel to places low on food and be scared to turn out for summer.

Gain support from the mentor or administrator if necessary. Look back on how you have built the relationship deeply when misbehavior moments begin at the end of the year. Do not just go through the motions—work toward prioritizing and inspiring as many students as possible in the final days. The new teacher will be frazzled and flustered with a million things to do—keep a check-off list and learn to prioritize. Remember that everything will get done one step at a time. Focus on the relationships to the bitter end.

Take advantage of ways to continue to impact lives. You understand this may be the last chance before summer. What is the need of each student? See it—focus on it—live in the now. Focus on material and do not get overwhelmed. Try not to finish too early before school ends.

Keep students busy and inform parents of all end-of-school activities. Work to send parents off with one final word of optimism to show how much you care about the student and the parent connections. Work on an organization and complete the lists. Check off items and begin to plan organization and changes for next year. Get in the correct mindset to enjoy the end. Soon you will be relaxing on vacation.

Make sure you can look back and say, *"job well done."* Remaining in the positive circle will impact everything one does in the final days. Chip in and support the team with any last-minute needs. The time has come; how will you choose this moment in time? Unfortunately, the final days are just as hard as the beginning of the year. You must pack the room, complete all inventory, participate in field day, awards day, and one last goodbye.

The new teacher balance will be more crucial than ever. Decisions and multi-tasking will be at the highest level of the year. Utilize the strategies learned throughout the year to take care of yourself. Try and stop and reflect as much as possible.

Reflections:

- What is the specific plan to finish strong?
- From whom do you need support to finish the year?
- When you feel you cannot go on, how will you travel to the belief and reframe it for success?
- How, when you want to give up, will you choose the power of can?

STORY TIME

A new teacher reflected on the end of her first year of teaching. She stated that every day was becoming more difficult to finish strong. Finally, she decided to begin a project with students to give back to the community. They collected food for a pantry nearby the school. She was astonished that it provided the feeling of gratitude that the entire classroom needed to finish the year feeling accomplished and taking the pity off herself.

Chapter 25

The Last Hour: Now What?

The last hour has arrived and it is time to process feelings. The students will respond with comments like "I do not want to leave you." In your mind, you will be thinking the same thing. The teacher realizes they have spent the entire year growing, learning, and laughing together. The new teacher reflects and has a proper understanding that they worked and became a true family. Yet, now somehow, it is time to let them go.

Unfortunately, some educators might not be prepared for when the last student walks out of the classroom for summer, the room is empty, and the lights go out. The new educator will be experiencing many different emotions. It may begin to consume the new teacher after completing the first year of teaching. It is likely that tears or maybe even sobbing will begin to occur. Do not be alarmed; this will all be part of the separation process.

Some will be engulfed in sadness, happiness, exhaustion, anticipation, and a sense of nervousness, to name a few. Some will continue embarking through emotions in the next month or two. However, many will not understand the process until the following year.

A particular type of mourning over the first group of students will occur. It is a process that will be draining *but necessary*. The educator will feel they will never love or be close to another group of students in the same way. However, one will find that each group is unique, and happiness and excitement will occur again; it is promised. However, it may be in a different manner each year. Planning a lengthy career in education, one might never get used to this painful process; acceptance will be necessary.

Every single year will be an experience of different personalities and different understandings. It will always be a new challenge, and the educator will be ready to travel that journey next August. So, take heart and let the summer be a time of healing, reflection, and growing in the profession.

Find ways to celebrate and replenish the spirit. You have many things to be proud of after the first year. Give the mind the peace it needs and gain the rest that the body is craving. Take into account everything learned and practiced, the reflection will begin to occur naturally. Choose a professional plan and set goals later in the summer after taking care of yourself and feeling in the right mindset for growth. It will be hectic when returning, but the new teacher will have a year under the belt and be more prepared.

Reflections:

- How will you be good to yourself over the summer?
- In what ways will continued growth of the craft of teaching be exhibited?
- In reflecting on the year, what changes are needed to become a better teacher?

STORY TIME

A new teacher reflected on emotions, as the award ceremony was happening on the last day of school. She could barely talk as tears flooded her face. She hugged the last child, and a parent came up to her who had been difficult throughout the year. The gentleman told her that she ended up being the best teacher her son had ever had. She knew at that moment, in front of everyone, she had chosen the correct profession.

Chapter 26

Final Thoughts

The most successful teachers all have a unique quality. They can stay positive through it all. Their positive energy affects others, and as a result, they are more effective in teaching and influencing behaviors. Things seem effortless for them. They have more patience and empathy. They smile more and take better care of themselves physically, mentally, and emotionally.

Positivity is not an inherited trait. It takes a bit of conscious effort, but anyone can learn to be positive with a few simple techniques. Positivity will give a person faith in their abilities, other people, and the belief that everything will work out as it should. Positive energy is like a force that surrounds a person, and it will heal those all around. We call this force field the positive circle.

Always embrace your potential, purpose, and passion. Commit, and you will never regret the choice. Stay focused on relationships, growth, and resilience in the journey. Set the goal to be a positive teacher and positive influence on everyone in the district. Remember, teachers will always matter in the positive circle. Now stand up, look in the mirror at your reflection, set positive intentions, and get on the mark, get set, go!

New teachers celebrate; you have made so much progress.

- "I am interested in progress, not perfection. Don't tell me; show me!"—Jennifer Limerick
- "Perfect classrooms get loud and a little messy sometimes!" "Consistency is secret to a safe environment." "Take your breaks!"—Kate Barton
- "More teenagers are working and focused on earning an income to help support themselves and their families than we realize."—April Dudynski
- "Anything worth having never comes easy, don't give up!"—Autumn Dove
- "Black and Brown students are fighting to be truly seen. They are hurting and are tired."—April Dudynski

Table 26.1 Final Reflections

Please rate the first year in the classroom on a scale from 1 to 10	1 2 3 4 5 6 7 8 9 10 Notice and Reflections
Relationships exist between teams, administrators, and school employees. In the reflection list examples of ways that enhanced these relationships. The new teacher grew in engagement in dialogue with correct feedback and it reflects a respect for diverse ideas that lead to further growth. In the reflection list specific feedback examples. Did the new teacher meet the goal set for the year by the administrator? In the reflection list the examples. Did the new teacher develop a plan for teacher growth? In the reflection list the classes taken. How engaged were the students in the classroom throughout the school year? In the reflection list ways that showed.	

- "You control you. And you should never give that control to someone else."—Amanda Oliver
- "Advocacy is important to this generation, and they want to know more about how to do it effectively."—April Dudynski
- "There is a powerful but true African proverb which states, *It takes a village to raise a child*. With this proverb in mind one can say, *It takes a village to grow a teacher*. Whether you are in year 1 or 21, all teachers and administrators can grow and learn from one another. Early on in my teaching career I made many mistakes in this profession. I think it is extremely important to give yourself permission to fail. As a teacher you must have resilience and humility. Don't be afraid to ask your colleague or an administrator for help. In addition, be vulnerable by sharing your past failures with inexperienced teachers and colleagues. By doing

so you can give them valuable tools to help them navigate through their current or future challenges."—Andre Long
- "Teenagers are looking for answers. They think it's a diagnosis, and maybe they do want that, but they are deeply searching to understand why they feel what they feel and respond how they respond."—April Dudynski

Epilogue

Once I entered into marriage and had children, career reflections occurred, and I decided to reanalyze my traveling decisions. For a while, I pondered the "why" of my occupation. I reflected on my love of children and how I could possibly make an impact on education. Initially hired at a high socio-economic school teaching third grade, I was introduced to a dynamic team and, in the first year, proudly provided with a lot of resources and helpful words of wisdom. I found teaching strategically compliant students with a lot of background experience rewarding for the first five years.

The most challenging element was finding ways to challenge these students and keep them excited about learning. My perspective changed in many ways over the next few years. First, I tried to find ways to reach students. Then, having an "a-ha moment" and finding something exciting—all kids want to be loved. Finally, I realized in my makeup that it came easy to share the love.

Great memories flow over from this school. Every day was a new adventure with children. One morning when my class was coming in from P.E., we were trying to find our seats. A small boy shouts: "my friend is vomiting!" It was everywhere as we began trying to scurry children out the door, take care of the sick child, and regain composure because the expensive shoes were now carrying vomit. Wow! No one warned me how to plan for this experience.

While teaching a section on the pioneer days, I thought it would be appropriate and educational to watch *Little House on the Prairie* one day with my 3rd graders. It turns out this was the episode that Ma Ingalls had a baby! So the pioneer lesson quickly and unexpectedly turned to a lesson on the birds and the bees! Lesson to learn the hard way—*always* preview a video.

Halfway into my fifth year, my dad passed away, and my world changed forever. His passing was the most devastating thing that ever happened in my life, and I soon realized it would take little effort to hunker down in my bed and never get up again. Knowing the need for a change, my family decided to move to where my husband grew up: Alaska. I was able to get a job quickly in second grade, which was not a massive transition from third grade. I soon found out that the difference in schools was the small-town feel. Instead of the hundred-dollar spa gift cards for Christmas, I received delicious homemade moose sausage. I enjoyed getting to know a new culture and how things worked, including the snow and moose on the playground.

Jump ahead a few years, and my daughter graduated from high school. I wondered why my mother had not warned me about how devastating this experience would be. I remember the day my husband, son, and I all headed to the airport to send her off to the university thousands of miles away. My husband would be the one to fly out and help my daughter move into the dorm since I would be starting the school year and unable to travel with them.

I attempted to begin to drive home from the airport in complete tears. Then suddenly, my son looked at me and, crying, said, "Mom, you know it will never be the same again." I finally had to ask him to stop talking so I could drive us safely. In the meantime, my daughter, who was crying in the airport, was approached by a stranger who consoled her, thinking she was suffering from the death of a loved one. Anyone who has experienced this significant family change knows how dramatic this change can be when your child heads to college out of state.

So, I decided again I needed change. I told my principal I wanted to teach kindergarten. She looked at me as though I was crazy. Thankfully, she granted my wish. It was like magic when I entered the room. You could feel the love of these young children. One little girl was telling me how pretty I was and how excited they all were about school. This experience was terrific, having twenty-four young children hanging on every word that comes out of your mouth!

One story in particular comes to mind. When the movie *Frozen* came out, a little girl asked me if I had seen it. I replied "no." Then, she asked if I could play the song "Let It Go" for the class. Suddenly, every boy and girl looked like they were in a musical dancing and singing around the classroom. There was never a dull moment in this classroom. Some of the challenges included getting an entire class into snowsuits to travel outside to play in the darkness, only to return inside to take it all off and hang up wet clothes. We lived in a valley and would receive hurricane-force winds periodically. My very first terrifying experience began when I had barely arrived at school.

I ran to my principal's office and asked where our "safe place" was located. I looked at her with my big eyes, and in my southern voice, I shouted, "We need to hunker down!" I will never forget how she looked at my face and laughed. I realized I had only known her for a couple of months, but she seemed pretty lovely, and I had grown to respect her quite quickly. My first thought was she had also lost it due to the high winds. Then, my mind began to think, okay, *you* might have to support *her* today. I was thinking about going into emergency mode. Then, in a very calm voice, after the laughing diminished, she stated, "This is normal."

Epilogue

One October afternoon, one of my small kindergarten students got picked up by the wind, and another teacher caught her from blowing away. I was terrified and thought, okay, nothing ordinary about this weather. I was in disbelief of how this could be anywhere close to normal. But I soon realized this was "Alaska normal."

The last surviving kindergarten story was the day I had a sub. I was actually in the building for a meeting. The substitute evidently did not see my clipboard with all the names for transportation on how students were getting home. He pulled my poster from the first day of school off the wall and placed students on different buses.

Luckily, most students knew what bus they were to get on to travel home. Except for one student who decided that it would be fun to get on the swim bus. We had an after-school program in which students who were signed up could travel to a pool by bus and participate in swimming class. This one child had told me many times about how she wanted to be a part of that class. Well, that day, she took it upon herself to attend.

I got a phone call in the office from her mother. She was panicked because her daughter did not arrive home and her grandpa was waiting. I began to call the bus barn, alarmed at where my five-year-old student had gone. The swim bus reported she was at the pool. I called her mom back and told her I had found her. Mom was about an hour away, so I told her I would get the student and bring her home. I arrived at the pool to see my student in a swimsuit and swimming in the pool. She was waving at me, having the time of her life. I panicked again, thinking how there was no permission for any of this. The lifeguard got her out of the pool and proceeded to tell me her clothes were in the dryer because they got wet. I had to wait at the pool for another forty-five minutes while they dried.

Then I had to drive her forty minutes home to her grandpa. The entire way, my student was saying how much fun the day was and how much she liked my truck. I told her how terrified her mom was and how this could never happen again. When we arrived, I sat and tried to calm her grandpa down. I finally came home around 7:30 pm that evening. I was exhausted and knew it was another story for the book.

The Alaska teaching adventure lasted five years. During this time, I would fall many times on the shiny ice. I survived the 75-mph winds in the dead of winter where literally "freezing one's face off" is a reality. I finally told my husband I needed to travel back to my Texas roots before I broke a hip on the ice, never to recover again. I had thought I wanted to go back to my previous school, which was a safe bet. However, I received a divine message to travel to a town I had only traveled through once in my early childhood. Somehow, the Lord had a different plan for me.

I would teach at a low socioeconomic Title 1 school in which I did not know anyone. It was a small-town atmosphere, but characteristics emulated more urban-like demographics. The students suffered from learning gaps created through generational poverty. Individually, each student had unique areas of assets and challenges. My assigned role for the campus would be teaching fourth grade reading/writing and social studies. The challenges that faced me for the next year would change my life forever and prove a mission and purpose.

I soon discovered that not even the basic needs of these children were anywhere near met. They would come to school hungry and tired from sleeping on the floor. I was the only consistent, safe thing in some of their daily lives. I remember one day having a simple bag of Cheez-Its on my desk when a student wanted to ask me a question. In a very soft voice, he said, "Are those Cheez-Its?" I replied "yes," and he said, "Wow, I have never had those but always wanted to try them." The next day, I had a box of Cheez-Its waiting for him to enjoy. You would have thought it was a filet mignon or fresh lobster tail. Simple—but life-changing in a young boy's life.

Some would come to school with bites from bed bugs, bruises from abuse, and bags under their eyes from no sleep. I understood where I belonged and knew this would be the most challenging next few years of my life. I experienced students lying, cheating, stealing, and talking back. The stories could go on and on, but above all, the one thing they all needed was love and a relationship with someone who genuinely cared and would keep them safe. I soon realized this relationship component was imperative and without it, no one would become educated. I understood these students wanted to feel safe and loved more than anything. I again could provide both very easily.

So, I began my journey of trying to change lives positively. I wanted to be the light that shined for them daily. I worked on building a relationship with one child at a time. It was not easy because I looked and acted differently. Nevertheless, I knew I had a heart full of grit in which I was not going to give up. Even today, as I drive to this sleepy little town, I am reminded of the purpose I have in pouring my heart and soul into this school district. I will always strive to have everyone join the positive circle.

Bibliography

Covey, Stephen M. R. "How the Best Leaders Build Trust." LeadershipNow, 2002. Accessed May 1, 2021. https://www.leadershipnow.com/CoveyOnTrust.html.

Goodpaster, Kasey P., Omolola A. Adedokun, and Gabriela C. Weaver. "Teachers' Perceptions of Rural Stem Teaching: Implications for Rural Teacher Retention." *The Rural Educator* 33, no. 3 (2018): 9–22. https://doi.org/10.35608/ruraled.v33i3.408.

Hattie, John, and Helen Timperley. "The Power of Feedback." *Review of Educational Research* 77, no. 1 (March 2007): 81–112. https://doi.org/10.3102/003465430298487.

"The Glossary of Education Reform." The Glossary of Education Reform. Accessed July 5, 2021. https://www.edglossary.org/.

McCullough, Michael E., Robert A. Emmons, and Jo-Ann Tsang. "Penn Institute Gratitude Questionnaire: Social Skills Plus." *Social Skills Plus*. Accessed November 10, 2021. https://socialskillsplus.com/wp-content/uploads/2018/11/Penn-Institute-Gratitude-Questionnaire.pdf.

About the Author

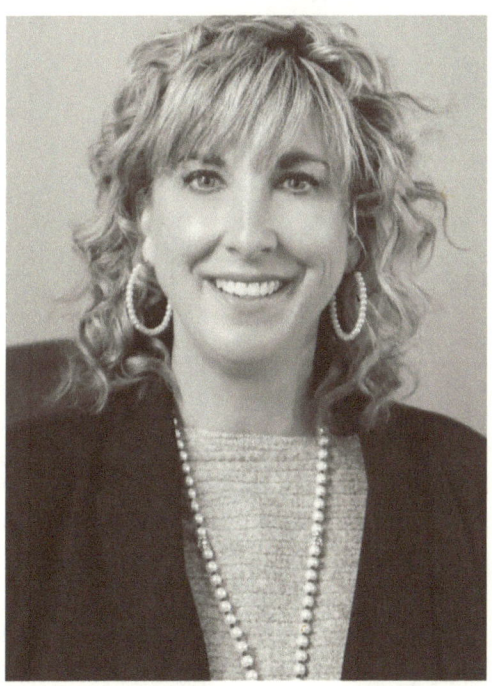

Julie West has been a Texas-based consummate and professional educator for seventeen years. She works as a literacy blended learning coach and a reading academy cohort leader for the Terrell Independent School District. She collaborates with educators and school administrators to improve the curriculum and increase student learning and achievement. Additionally, she offers personalized professional development, working closely with all teachers. Prior to becoming a part of the curriculum and instruction team, she was a classroom teacher for fifteen years. Julie helped create a new teacher academy for her current district to retain new educators. She attended Texas A&M University–Commerce, graduating with a master's degree in Reading Instruction.

www.ingramcontent.com/pod-product-compliance
Lightning Source LLC
Chambersburg PA
CBHW032028230426
43671CB00005B/241